Nearly 70 Million Americans Rely on Medicare and Medicaid

- 36 million senior citizens and disabled Americans receive Medicare. The program is divided into two parts: Part A covers hospital costs, and Part B covers doctors costs.

- 33 million needy Americans of all ages receive Medicaid.

Medicare and Medicaid Need Help

- Spending on Medicare and Medicaid will double every five to seven years.

- Medicare Part A was originally expected to cost $9.1 billion in 1990. It actually cost $66.6 billion.

- Medicaid was supposed to cost $1 billion in 1990. It actually cost $92 billion.

- According to the Medicare Trustees, Medicare Part A may go bankrupt in the year 2002 or sooner.

- Today, there are approximately four workers for every person receiving Medicare. In less than fifty years, there will be about two workers for every Medicare participant.

WE MUST SOLVE THESE PROBLEMS NOW!

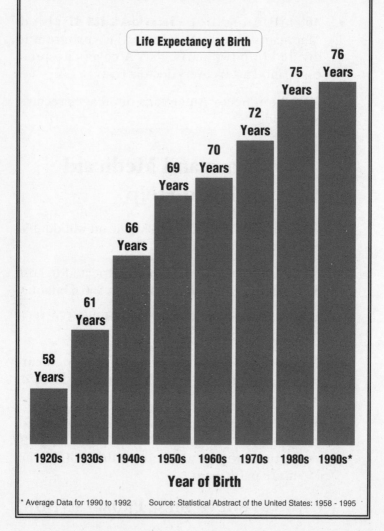

Thanks to health care advances, Americans are living longer today than ever before.

The challenge now is to pay for our success.

Life Expectancy at Birth

76 Years

75 Years

72 Years

70 Years

69 Years

66 Years

61 Years

58 Years

1920s 1930s 1940s 1950s 1960s 1970s 1980s 1990s*

Year of Birth

INTENSIVE CARE

We Must Save Medicare and Medicaid Now

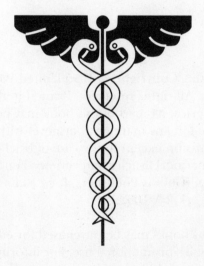

ROSS PEROT

■ HarperPerennial
A Division of HarperCollins*Publishers*

HarperCollins books may be purchased for educational, business, or sales promotional use. For information please write: Special Markets Department, HarperCollins Publishers, Inc., 10 East 53rd Street, New York, NY 10022.

FIRST EDITION

ISBN 0-06-095172-9

95 96 97 98 99 RRD 10 9 8 7 6 5 4 3 2 1

CONTENTS

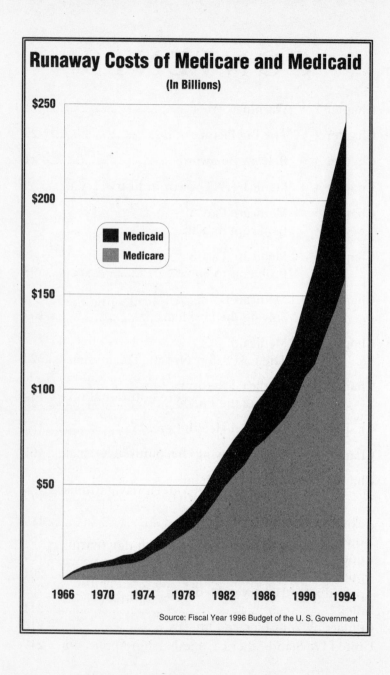

Runaway Costs of Medicare and Medicaid
(In Billions)

Source: Fiscal Year 1996 Budget of the U. S. Government

1

Warning Lights

The year is 1995, and you are a passenger on an airliner. This particular airplane shows signs of aging because it has not been overhauled in the 30 years since it was built. The equipment is old and out of date, which makes it difficult to navigate and fly the aircraft. To compensate for these deficiencies, the cockpit has been expanded to include the first class section where additional pilots and navigators are advising the flight crew.

Many technological advances have occurred since the plane was manufactured in 1965. Sandwich-size computers in newer airplanes can plot a course and make adjustments instantaneously. Modern navigation systems can locate an aircraft anywhere in the world within three feet.

Instead of having these modern-day features, the cabin of your plane is lined with various dials, gauges, and warning lights. All eyes are glued to the instruments. You're beginning to feel uneasy about the situation, but you have no choice in the matter. At 35,000 feet, you're committed.

INTENSIVE CARE

Suddenly, everything seems to go wrong. The dials are spinning wildly and the warning lights are lit up like a pinball machine. The crew members are shouting, but the advice is confusing and inconsistent. The plane is beginning to lose altitude. No one seems to be in charge. Decisive action is needed quickly to avoid tragedy.

Today, America's health care programs for senior citizens and the needy are approaching the same situation. If measures are not taken now to repair these important programs, they too will begin to break down and cause problems for everyone involved in the health care industry, especially the elderly and needy. The charts and graphs contained in this book are equivalent to the gauges and warning lights on the instrument panel of an airplane. They keep us informed about our surroundings, and they alert us to danger. This book will analyze the warning signals coming from those charts and graphs.

Like an airplane that is low on fuel, Medicare is running out of money. Like an old airplane that is too expensive to operate, both Medicare and Medicaid are straining the financial resources of our nation. If our elected leaders are ever going to make the tough decisions necessary to balance the budget, then these two health care programs will have to be updated. However, reforming Medicare and Medicaid *does not* necessarily mean reducing services. This book will devote a great deal of attention to the subject of alternative methods of paying for health care.

Like our airplane, Medicare and Medicaid were created in the mid-1960s. The primary objective of each of these programs was to assure senior citizens and the needy that they could obtain affordable, quality health care. The programs have been very successful in meeting these goals. The problem is that the costs were severely underestimated. In 1965, lawmakers had no way of knowing that the costs of these programs would reach the levels they are at today. This book will carefully examine these costs so that everyone can better understand why reform is desperately needed.

If the United States can put men on the moon and bring them back, then surely we can figure out how to save and improve Medicare and Medicaid. It must be done to preserve health care for the sake of the people who truly need it while improving the financial strength of our nation for our children.

The warning lights are flashing. Some of them are brighter than others, but they all relate to the condition of the airplane. We will have to deal with each of the warning lights — many of them at the same time — to save the passengers.

WARNING: MEDICARE & MEDICAID

Federal spending on the Medicare and Medicaid programs will total $267 billion in 1995. This will account for over 17% of the entire federal budget for the year. **THE COMBINED FEDERAL SPENDING ON MEDICARE AND MEDICAID COSTS AMERICA'S TAXPAYERS MORE THAN $30 MILLION EVERY HOUR OF EVERY DAY OF THE YEAR.**

If Medicare and Medicaid costs are not controlled, the quality of care these programs provide to nearly 70 million Americans will diminish considerably. Our government can never turn its back on Americans who need help. But the form of help that the government will *be able* to provide may be different than the level of help that is currently available.

Given the current political climate in Washington, updating the Medicare program and the Medicaid program is a virtual certainty. There is almost no argument in Congress about whether the budget should be balanced. The only discussion centers around the time required to reach a balanced budget (seven years vs. ten years) and whether or not a tax cut will be included in the plan. No tax increases are being proposed for the purpose of balancing the budget.

If no tax increases are planned, the only possible conclusion for the spending side of the budget equation is this: some previously scheduled spending increases for certain programs will have to be scaled back. The large amount of federal spending dedicated to Medicare and Medicaid guarantees the budgets for these programs will be examined closely.

In addition to the current size of these two programs, the other problem with Medicare and Medicaid is their past and projected growth rates.

FOR EXAMPLE, IN 1991 THE ONE-YEAR INCREASE IN MEDICAID SPENDING WAS 27%.

This was an unusual year, but there is nothing to prevent a similar occurrence in the future.

UNDER CURRENT CONDITIONS MEDICARE AND MEDICAID SPENDING ARE PROJECTED TO DOUBLE EVERY FIVE TO SEVEN YEARS.

This warning light has been flashing bright red for years, but it has been ignored by Washington. The chart on page 5 shows how quickly Medicare and Medicaid expenditures are anticipated to increase.

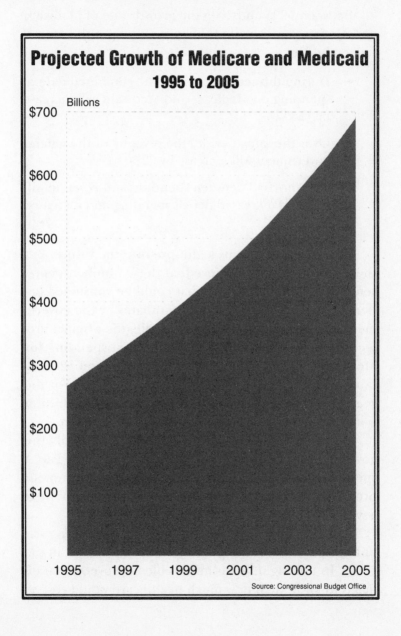

Projected Growth of Medicare and Medicaid
1995 to 2005

Billions

$700

$600

$500

$400

$300

$200

$100

1995   1997   1999   2001   2003   2005

Source: Congressional Budget Office

INTENSIVE CARE

Between 1995 and 2005 the growth rate of Medicare and Medicaid will exceed the growth rate of the overall federal budget.

- During this ten-year period the combined federal spending on Medicare and Medicaid will increase by 158%.

- Over the same period, the revenue of the federal government will increase by 62%.

- The shortfall between spending and revenue will result in increased deficit spending and increased debt.

These figures give us a glimpse into the future. But there is no reason to believe that these numbers represent the maximum amount that could be consumed under these programs. Spending estimates by the government are notoriously low. For example, the original projections prepared in 1965 estimated that spending for Medicare Part A for the year 1967 would total $2.3 billion. The actual amount spent was $3.4 billion. For the year 1990, the government estimated that $9.1 billion would be spent; the actual amount was $66.6 billion.

The chart on page 7 illustrates just how badly the government underestimated the original Medicare Part A spending projections. Like so many other government programs, Medicare and Medicaid took on a life of their own and began to expand without restraint.

The growth in Medicare and Medicaid spending was unimaginable when the programs were developed in the 1960s. In hindsight, it was impossible for government officials to know then how much health care would cost 30 years later. How can we be certain that we are any better today at forecasting 30 years ahead to the year 2025?

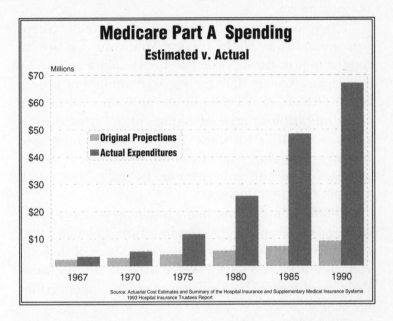

Technological advances in the field of medicine have improved health care and increased life expectancy. The average American today will live more than five years longer than the average American in 1965.

WITH ALMOST 70 MILLION PEOPLE RELYING ON MEDICARE AND MEDICAID TODAY, THIS FIVE-YEAR IN-CREASE IN LIFE EXPECTANCY RESULTS IN AN EXTRA 345 MILLION YEARS OF HEALTH CARE THAT MUST BE PAID FOR BY THE FEDERAL GOVERNMENT.

In addition to unforeseen advances in technology, other factors have contributed to the steep increases in the cost of the Medicare and Medicaid programs. Inflation, triggered by the oil shocks of 1973 and 1979, is certainly one cause that could not have been predicted. Another problem that was not easily foreseen is the amount of waste, fraud, and abuse that would occur within the two programs.

It is an unfortunate fact of life that dishonesty creeps into systems like Medicare and Medicaid that are intended to provide important services to older and needy Americans. But anytime such a large number of people are involved in such a complicated and expensive system, the temptation to take advantage of the situation becomes irresistible for some. People who are otherwise honest get caught up in a system where the only "victim" appears to be the government. **IN FACT, THE FINAL VICTIMS ARE THE TAXPAYERS.**

Billions of dollars are being lost every year as a result of illegal or deceptive practices by insurers, patients, doctors, and other health care providers. Much of this corrupt conduct could be uncovered with improved systems that detect unusual billing patterns and fraudulent claims for benefits.

The U.S. General Accounting Office, the federal government's financial watchdog agency, has determined that for every dollar spent to control fraud, the government saves about $14. Medicare is currently in the process of designing a computer system that should help combat waste, fraud, and abuse. The system, however, is at least three years away from completion.

Medicare and Medicaid must be updated to be as cost effective as possible. The federal government has been careless with the money it receives from America's hard-working taxpayers. Over the years, our elected leaders have allowed our nation to accumulate almost $5 *trillion* in debt.

WARNING LIGHTS

WARNING: THE DEBT

Our elected leaders have ignored the clear signals that the greatest nation in the history of man has been spending itself toward bankruptcy. The brightest warning light on the instrument panel reads NATIONAL DEBT. This light has been flashing for years, but few in Washington have taken it seriously.

In 1980, four years after the United States celebrated its 200th birthday, the national debt was $909 billion. Now, just 15 years later, the national debt is almost $5 trillion. This situation is unthinkable, yet this is where we find ourselves today.

The growth of the national debt has gone unchecked. Spending beyond our means has become an addiction. Members of Congress and presidents switched on the debt auto pilot and fell asleep at the controls. Years of indifference at the federal level have left us in serious danger. **NO OTHER NATION IN THE HISTORY OF MAN HAS EVER ACCUMULATED SO MUCH DEBT.** If no solutions are found soon, the national debt will swell to inconceivable proportions.

The chart on page 10 shows the growth of the federal debt. At the end of the most recent fiscal year (September 30, 1994), the total debt was $4,643,711,000,000. In simple terms, just think of it as the balance on a gigantic VISA or MasterCard account. It represents the difference between how much the government has spent and how much cash the government has collected in taxes and other revenues.

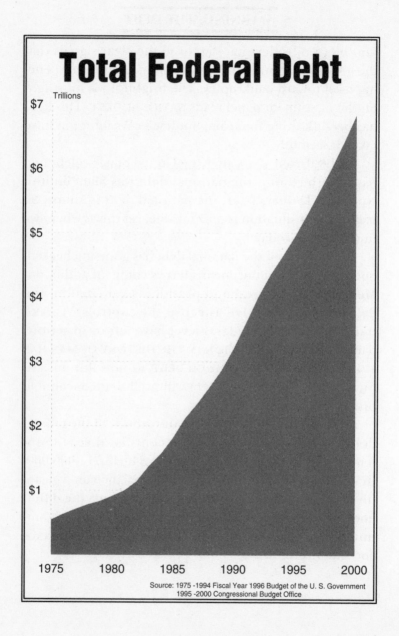

Total Federal Debt

Trillions

Source: 1975 -1994 Fiscal Year 1996 Budget of the U. S. Government
1995 -2000 Congressional Budget Office

WARNING LIGHTS

This chart also indicates that the debt is projected to rise to approximately $6.8 trillion by the end of this decade. That amount represents approximately $24,838 for every American, or $99,352 for a family of four. Again, to use simple terms, just think of it as mailing a credit card bill with a balance due of almost $25,000 plus interest to every single person in the country in the year 2000.

Congress and the White House must work together to pass a balanced budget. All of us must realize that balancing the budget can only be accomplished with a fair, shared sacrifice by every American. If we don't balance the budget, the national debt will continue to increase and it will exhaust America's financial strength.

Always remember that we, the American people, are the owners of this great nation. The national debt is our debt. Is it fair for us to ask our children and grandchildren to pay this debt for us? Left unchecked, the burden of the national debt will destroy the American Dream.

WARNING: THE DEFICIT

Each year during the budget debate, Congress and the President decide how much money the federal government will spend during the next fiscal year. If taxes and other revenues will exceed expenditures, the government is said to be *running a surplus* for that particular year. On the other hand, *deficit spending* occurs when the government spends more than the total of taxes and other revenue for that year. The United States has not had a budget surplus since 1969. The reason we have a national debt is that our deficits have been larger than our surpluses. **IN PLAIN TALK, WE SPEND MORE THAN WE RECEIVE.**

INTENSIVE CARE

The vast majority of Americans work hard every day and are able to make ends meet. Those who are disciplined, put money into savings. Year after year families cannot spend more money than they earn. Sooner or later the bill collectors will show up. Our elected leaders surely balance their family budgets. Now they need to apply the same principles to the national budget.

Just because we haven't had a balanced budget in 26 years doesn't mean that it isn't important to talk about having one. During election years, some political candidates notice the warning lights and talk about the problems facing our nation. Once in office, however, their appetite to make tough decisions becomes compromised by the need to get reelected. The easiest course of action for a politician is to ignore the warning lights and hope that something happens to make the problems go away. Problems are seldom solved without hard work, however. Ignoring them now usually makes them worse.

During the 1992 presidential election, Bill Clinton and Al Gore saw the warning lights, and promised to scale back deficit spending. In their campaign book, *Putting People First*, they stated:

> *Our plan will cut the deficit in half within four years and assure that it continues to fall each year after that. ... Never again should we pass on our debts to our children while their futures silently slip through our fingers.*

During his first year in office, President Clinton was able to reduce the size of the deficit. With a combination of tax increases, lower interest rates on the national debt, and targeted spending cuts, his first budget eliminated more than $50 billion from the $290 billion deficit during the last year of the Bush Administration. During the first year of the Clinton Administration, the federal budget was headed in the right direction for a change, and the gauges on the financial instrument panel looked a little better. It did not take long for politics-as-usual to get in the way of common sense.

The Clinton Administration did not have the discipline to maintain the same pace of reduction in the following years. Otherwise, their goal of cutting the deficit in half by 1997 could have been achieved. The problem, of course, was that in order to reduce the deficit in his first budget, President Clinton had to abandon his campaign promise for a middle-class tax cut. A tax cut would have only made the deficit worse. He then imposed the largest tax increase in history. Increased tax revenue helped to reduce the deficit.

When President Clinton prepared his second budget, there were only three choices for achieving further deficit reduction: cut spending, raise taxes on the middle class, or a combination of the two. Because none of these alternatives was politically acceptable, reducing annual deficit spending automatically fell off the Administration's radar screen.

The chart on page 14 illustrates that President Clinton's campaign promise "to cut the deficit in half within four years" was not kept. If the promise had been kept, annual deficit spending would be approximately $145 billion when his term ends in 1997. Instead, the President's Office of Management and Budget forecasts that deficit spending will remain or exceed the $200 billion level each year through the year 2000.

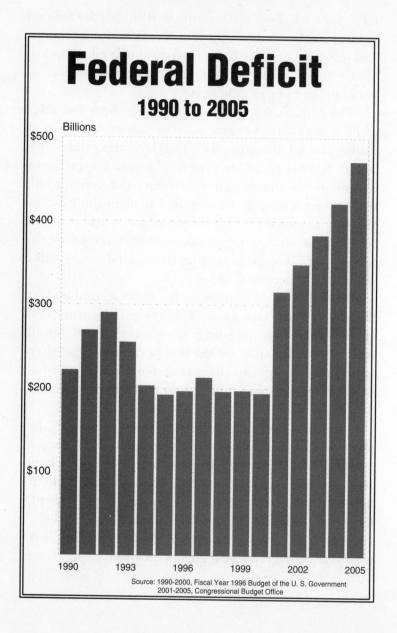

Federal Deficit
1990 to 2005

Billions

Source: 1990-2000, Fiscal Year 1996 Budget of the U. S. Government
2001-2005, Congressional Budget Office

WARNING LIGHTS

Congress has its own staff that handles budget-related matters. The Congressional Budget Office (CBO) prepares a separate projection of deficit spending. This projection is more pessimistic than that of the Administration. The chart on page 14 indicates the CBO believes that deficit spending will be $316 billion in 2001 and rise to $472 billion by 2005.

Even assuming the more optimistic numbers from the White House, another $1 trillion would be added to the federal debt before the end of this decade. Can the United States of America afford to begin the 21st century almost $7 trillion in debt? NO!

If this news is not bad enough, the White House itself predicts that it will only get worse — much worse — in the long run. Alice Rivlin, President Clinton's budget director, wrote a memo in October 1994 titled "Big Choices."

In her memo, Ms. Rivlin presented President Clinton and his staff with forecasts made by the Office of Management and Budget. The chart on page 16 is truly frightening.

Ms. Rivlin's data indicates that by the year 2020, the deficit spending for that year alone will be more than $1.4 trillion. *This is an amount that is almost equal to the entire federal budget for 1995.* Ten years later, in 2030, annual deficit spending is projected to exceed $4 trillion. Remember, *this is the amount of money that will be added to the debt in just one year.*

With the Republican party capturing control of Congress in the November 1994 elections, the President's party no longer solely controls budgetary decisions. No matter which party controls Congress, the Republicans and Democrats can both see the same warning lights.

INTENSIVE CARE

Their job is to react wisely and swiftly and to deliver their passengers — the American people — safely to their destination. That destination is a future free from the burdens imposed by a crushing load of debt.

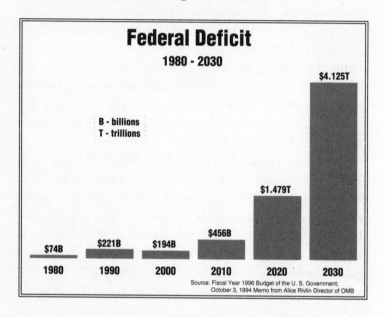

Federal Deficit

1980 - 2030

$4.125T

B - billions
T - trillions

$1.479T

$456B

$74B $221B $194B

1980   1990   2000   2010   2020   2030

Source: Fiscal Year 1996 Budget of the U. S. Government;
October 3, 1994 Memo from Alice Rivlin Director of OMB

WARNING: INTEREST PAYMENTS

Thus far we have talked about the twin problems of the debt and the deficit. The symptom of these problems is the enormous amount of interest paid each year on the national debt. It doesn't take an economist to understand what is happening: a persistent pattern of deficit spending increases the national debt, which results in higher and higher interest payments every year.

Interest on the national debt buys nothing for the people of the United States. It's like having a hole in the fuel tank of our airplane — we keep pumping money into the government, but part of it gets wasted. It is estimated that a total of $234 billion will be spent on interest for the fiscal year ending September 30, 1995. By comparison, a total of $267 billion is projected to be spent on Medicare and Medicaid for the same time period.

The chart below shows how the interest on the debt is rising. The government must pay this money every year. As interest payments rise, spending on other programs may be cut. Because of their size, Medicare and Medicaid could become prime targets. If spending cannot be cut, annual deficit spending will be increased, and the national debt will grow even larger.

Interest on the national debt can take money out of the pockets of taxpayers in more ways than one. First, income taxes remain higher than they should because of the required interest payments on the debt. Second, interest rates for everything else are higher than they oth-

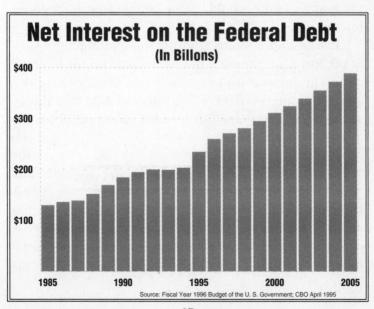

Net Interest on the Federal Debt
(In Billons)

Source: Fiscal Year 1996 Budget of the U. S. Government; CBO April 1995

erwise would be if the government were not competing for funds. It is the simple law of supply and demand — if the government did not need to borrow money, there would be less demand for funds and therefore a lower interest rate on loans for homes, cars and education.

For example, the two most expensive items that most people own are their homes and their automobiles. The biggest break that the federal government could give taxpayers is not a tax cut. Instead, the fastest way of saving money for most Americans is to give them a break on the amount of interest they pay on their homes and automobiles.

As of April 1995, the average home mortgage in the United States was $107,900 with an interest rate of 7.99%. If the interest rate declined by 25%, the annual mortgage payments would decline by about $1,500. The IRS reports that income taxes averaged $5,796 per taxpayer in 1993. Even if income tax rates could be cut by as much as 25%, the average family would still be better off with the lower interest rates.

If Washington keeps ignoring the warning lights such as the increasing amount of interest paid on the national debt, the federal fuel tank will run dry. Because the amount of interest paid on the national debt is so threatening to our economic future, we'll take another look at it in the next chapter.

WARNING: CHILDREN ON BOARD

During any discussion of the national debt and the government's addiction to deficit spending, a reference is usually made to the consequences they will have on future generations of Americans — and rightfully so. This book is no exception. If the national debt could be paid off by the same generation that incurred it, there wouldn't really be much to talk about.

There is nothing inherently wrong with a reasonable amount of debt. Our property laws and social policies encourage home ownership. Borrowing money for the purpose of buying a home is an accepted activity and it is vital to our economy. Most home mortgages are scheduled to be repaid in 30 years or less. This time period roughly coincides with the expected income-earning years of the borrowers at the time they decide to buy a home.

The point is that borrowing by homebuyers is unlike borrowing by the government. They are different in at least two ways. First, the purpose of government borrowing, for the most part, is to finance current consumption, whereas the purpose of a home mortgage is to construct an asset that will have financial value long after the debt has been repaid.

The second difference is that the responsibility for repaying the debt on a home can be assigned to a particular generation. Parents buy a home to raise their family. Under normal circumstances, the principal and interest gets paid during the working years of the parents, and they retire with no debt.

Unlike a home mortgage, when the government borrows money, it doesn't make principal payments on the debt. Instead, the government just pays interest — usually for one, five, ten, twenty, or thirty years — until the debt is due to be paid. At that time, the government simply borrows more money to pay back the first lender. In this way, the debt gets passed on to succeeding generations who had no voice in the decision. This resembles a pyramid scheme where the early investors get paid off with money raised from later investors.

The phrase "Passing the debt on to our children" is an abstract concept, until someone can say how much it will cost. Someone has done that, and his name is Dr. Laurence Kotlikoff. In his book, *Generational Accounting*, Dr. Kotlikoff relates current government spending practices to future tax rates.

Dr. Kotlikoff's work has been used by the Clinton Administration. On page 25 of the 1995 federal budget, it was stated that the next generation to be born will pay an 82% tax rate during their lifetime.

When President Clinton's 1996 budget was released, the generational accounting information had been omitted. Why? Two explanations are likely: (1) the tax rate on future generations had climbed to 84%; and/or (2) deficit reduction was no longer a priority for the Administration.

WARNING: LOW WAGES AHEAD

In theory, as a nation's economy grows so should its wages. Growing wages should result in an expanded tax base which, in turn, generates new revenue for the government. The growth in *real wages* has been relatively stagnant since 1965. The term *real wages* means wages as adjusted for the effects of inflation. It is a method of measuring the purchasing power of the dollar. A person earning $15,000 in 1965 would need to earn $63,056 in 1991 to have kept pace with inflation. If the same person had earned $55,000 in 1991, his purchasing power would have only been equivalent to $13,084 in 1965 dollars.

WARNING LIGHTS

Various factors have combined over the past 30 years to keep the growth of wages low in the United States. We have lost many of our good paying manufacturing jobs to our foreign competitors. This has forced much of our skilled and semi-skilled labor force to accept lower wages.

Another reason usually given for the sluggish growth of wages is the rising cost of health care. To attract qualified employees, most employers offer some type of health care coverage. Employers view the cost of health coverage as another form of compensation they pay to their employees. The fact that employers are paying more and more each year for health insurance coverage directly impacts their ability to increase wages. Even if an employee does not receive a regular salary increase, his or her overall compensation is actually increasing if the employer is providing health care coverage.

The graph on page 22 shows the growth of health care costs compared with wages since 1965. Health care benefits for employees have been growing out of control while real wages have grown only seven percent since 1965. This is not seven percent per year; it is seven percent over the entire period.

For an employee to believe that he or she does not pay for health insurance is wrong. The employee pays for it in the form of wages that could otherwise be higher if not for the burden of steadily increasing health care costs.

The graph on page 22 is one warning light that has not been ignored. Employers in the private sector began reacting to the signals of rapidly rising health care costs some time ago. This warning light was labeled NET PROFIT. Employers everywhere realized that something had to be done to control rapidly rising health care costs. They had to protect their bottom line.

The private sector has taken the lead in health care reform by proving that health care costs can be controlled without sacrificing quality or coverage. Many companies have given their employees a choice of different health care plans. This is perhaps the main reason that private sector health care costs are currently under control and even decreasing. In 1994, health care costs per private-sector employee actually decreased by one percent.

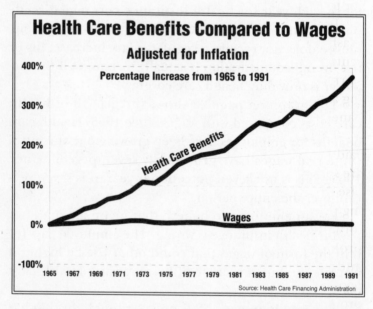

Health Care Benefits Compared to Wages

Source: Health Care Financing Administration

The measures taken by the private sector to control costs will be discussed later in this book. The important fact is that the private sector has taken effective steps to control health care expenses while preserving the quality of service. These plans can serve as a blueprint for the government to save the Medicare and Medicaid programs.

WE NEED ACTION THIS DAY

Whenever Winston Churchill wanted immediate action on an item, he would write the message, "Action this day," across a note or memorandum. Instead of using the Churchill approach, the government seems to be using the ostrich approach. It has buried its head in the sand and ignored the problems with Medicare and Medicaid for too many years.

Inaction on difficult issues is all too common in Washington. One of the unfortunate aspects of a representative form of government is that the representatives worry too much about getting reelected. Instead of looking at the polls, they should be watching the instrument panel.

The warning lights triggered by Medicare and Medicaid have been ignored for years because these programs are so politically sensitive. Most politicians want someone else to take the political risks associated with modernizing these programs. In the absence of someone stepping forward to take the risks, they continue to hope that the problems will disappear. The problems with Medicare and Medicaid need to be explained to the American people. The options that are available to modernize these programs must also be explained.

The American people are not adequately informed about the dangers created by our government's financial irresponsibility. This is partly the fault of our elected leaders and partly our own fault. If the owners of this country cannot get straight answers from Washington, we owe it to ourselves to take the initiative and find the answers. One of the main objectives of this book is to alert the American people to the harmful consequences that runaway deficit spending imposes on programs such as Medicare and Medicaid.

Our elected leaders will be much more likely to take action once the American people become aware of the uncertain financial future of Medicare and Medicaid. The voice of the voters is much stronger than warning lights.

AVOIDING DISASTER

Warning lights are flashing across the instrument panel of the federal government. The gauges on the instrument panel are also showing signs of danger. The two gauges marked MEDICARE and MEDICAID are rising exceptionally fast. The costs of both programs will be contributors to, as well as victims of, the impending disaster.

Medicare and Medicaid are going bankrupt before our eyes. As these programs consume larger portions of the federal budget, it will become even more difficult to balance the budget.

The chart on page 25 shows the portion of total federal spending that Medicare and Medicaid consume. As both programs continue to grow, they will take up a larger piece of the pie. Other large portions of the budget, such as Social Security and the interest on the debt, are also growing. They *must* also be paid each year by the government. The piece of the pie titled "domestic discretionary" is the money used to pay for federal programs such as education, agriculture, and housing. As

Medicare and Medicaid spending increases, this important piece of the budget is forced to become smaller.

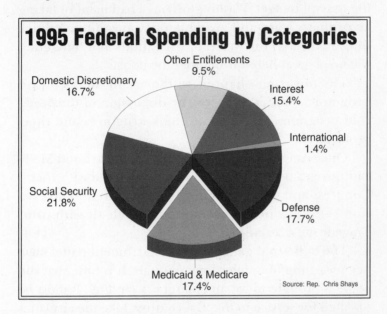

1995 Federal Spending by Categories

Other Entitlements
9.5%

Domestic Discretionary
16.7%

Interest
15.4%

International
1.4%

Social Security
21.8%

Defense
17.7%

Medicaid & Medicare
17.4%

Source: Rep. Chris Shays

A balanced budget will mean that the growth of large spending programs like Medicare and Medicaid must be controlled. The federal government clearly cannot continue on its current financial path. Our children and grandchildren deserve an economically sound nation. Today's senior citizens and needy individuals deserve quality health care. If Medicare and Medicaid are not modernized right away, neither will happen.

The key to saving these programs and the financial state of our great nation is understanding the issues surrounding Medicare and Medicaid. If we fail to understand the problems, we will never be able to arrive at a solution that is any better than the system we have today. Chapter 2 discusses these issues.

Chapter 3 will explain some unusual terminology that the government uses in connection with Medicare and the federal budget. Washington has a bad habit of taking an ordinary word and giving it a new meaning. A quick introduction to the world of trust funds and budgeting will be of great help throughout the book.

The next four chapters will focus on the Medicare program. Chapter 8 begins the discussion of the Medicaid program. We'll look at their structures and their problems.

Once Americans understand the Medicare and Medicaid programs and the problems associated with them, Congress and the President will be required to take action. This is a problem that must be dealt with now. Tragedy must be averted.

The lights and gauges on the instrument panel have been warning of danger long enough. It is time that the plane is brought in for an emergency landing. It must be updated for service in the 21st century. Like the airplanes of today, Medicare and Medicaid can be made more efficient and more economical while offering better service than the original model of 30 years ago.

2

The Big Picture

The pilot of an airplane in trouble usually doesn't have much time to react. Although the instrument panel will indicate which systems and components may be causing trouble, that may not be the complete story. Severe weather conditions, a wind shear for example, could be the source of the problem. In an emergency situation, the pilot must take into account both internal and external conditions when trying to decide what corrective measures to take.

Like our airplane, something is wrong with Medicare and Medicaid. We know what the problem is — the programs are too expensive. However, we don't know all of the reasons why. We are certain that problems inside the two programs need to be corrected. But it is also very likely that outside conditions are contributing to the excessive costs. These outside conditions, of course, are the same factors that contribute to the high cost of health care throughout the system. This book will examine some of those factors and discuss proposals for dealing with them.

INTENSIVE CARE

Finding quick and practical solutions to the internal problems of Medicare and Medicaid will not be easy. Finding solutions to the external problems that affect Medicare and Medicaid will be extraordinarily complicated. When the debate begins, powerful lobbyists and special interests will be fighting for control of our airplane.

PIECES OF THE PUZZLE

Before getting into the details of Medicare and Medicaid, it is helpful to understand how these two programs fit into the overall health care system in the United States. It is also helpful to understand how the entire health care system relates to the overall economy of the United States.

In 1993, the last full year for which data is available, approximately $898 billion was spent for health care of all types in the United States. This amount includes payments to hospitals, doctors, pharmacies, medical equipment suppliers, long-term care facilities, and just about anything else normally associated with the health care industry, including the cost to build hospitals and clinics. The $898 billion represents the total amount of money spent by the public sector (Medicare and Medicaid, for example) and the private sector (individuals and companies that provide employees and their families with medical insurance coverage, for example).

Health care spending is a large segment of the economy of the United States. Economists use the term *Gross Domestic Product* (GDP) to measure the annual economic output of a nation. Technically speaking, the three major

components of GDP are purchases by consumers, private
investment, and government spending.

During 1993, the GDP of the United States was
$6.377 trillion. This means that health care amounted to
14% of the entire economy of the United States in 1993.
The chart below illustrates the growth of total health care
costs from 1960 to 1993. It also illustrates the increasing
proportion of GDP that health care has consumed since
1960.

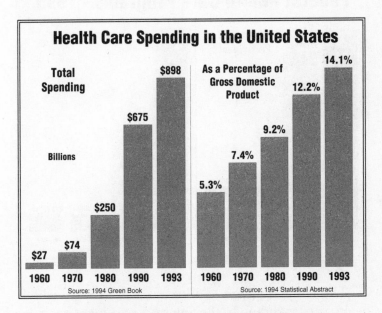

Health Care Spending in the United States

Total Spending — Billions

1960	1970	1980	1990	1993
$27	$74	$250	$675	$898

Source: 1994 Green Book

As a Percentage of Gross Domestic Product

1960	1970	1980	1990	1993
5.3%	7.4%	9.2%	12.2%	14.1%

Source: 1994 Statistical Abstract

FEDERAL HEALTH CARE PROGRAMS

As mentioned earlier, health care spending can be divided into two categories: the public sector and the private sector. The public sector (the federal government)
provides health care coverage to more than 86 million
people through several programs. The two largest federal

health care programs are Medicare and Medicaid. In addition, the federal government provides health care coverage to its employees, some of its retired employees who are not eligible for Medicare, and to retired members of the military. The following chart shows the number of individuals receiving benefits and the amount spent by these programs.

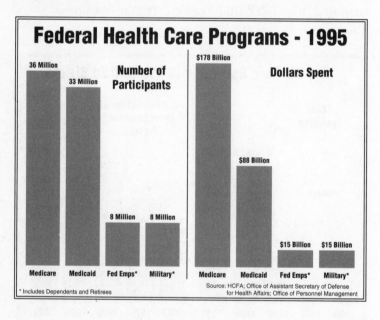

Federal Health Care Programs - 1995

Number of Participants

- Medicare: 36 Million
- Medicaid: 33 Million
- Fed Emps*: 8 Million
- Military*: 8 Million

* Includes Dependents and Retirees

Dollars Spent

- Medicare: $178 Billion
- Medicaid: $88 Billion
- Fed Emps*: $15 Billion
- Military*: $15 Billion

Source: HCFA; Office of Assistant Secretary of Defense for Health Affairs; Office of Personnel Management

The chart on page 31 illustrates the rate at which health care spending by the federal government has risen since 1965, the year Medicare and Medicaid were created. If no action is taken during the next few years, health care will be the largest category of government spending.

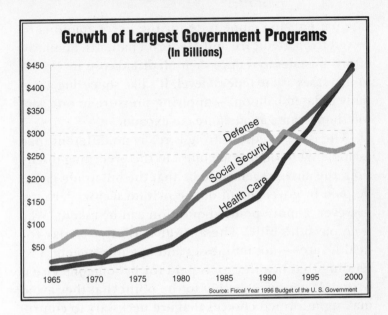

Growth of Largest Government Programs
(In Billions)

Source: Fiscal Year 1996 Budget of the U. S. Government

These projections assume that no additional benefits are added to the existing programs. If Congress decides to expand the number of people who are eligible for these federal programs, government spending for health care will grow even faster.

COST SHIFTING

One of the major problems in health care reform is the situation known as "cost shifting." In its search for ways to contain the rising costs of Medicare and Medicaid, Congress will be looking for ways to save money. The problem is that "savings" in one sector of the health care industry often become higher costs to another sector. For example, many measures to control costs in the Medicare program may result in increased costs to insurance companies as hospitals are forced to charge more to their private patients to compensate for the lower amounts received from Medicare and Medicaid patients. Similarly, efforts by states to reduce their Medicaid costs may result in increases at the federal level. It's like squeezing a partially inflated balloon — applying pressure in one spot will simply cause another area to expand.

The issue of cost shifting is really no different than asking, "Who will pay the bill?" In the preceding discussion, the answer seemed to be that the bill would either be paid by government or the private sector. Perhaps, however, a more pointed question can be asked: "Who *really* pays the bill?" The answer is that *people* pay for health care — not businesses and not government. Pretending that health care is paid for by someone else is wrong. It confuses people to the point that they avoid making informed choices that are necessary to control costs and keep health care affordable for everyone.

Not only is it wrong to pretend that health care is paid for by someone else, it is misleading to the hard working men and women of this country. Most employees are not aware of how much their employers pay for health insurance coverage. Actually, it is the employee who really pays for the health care coverage. This happens because health insurance is a form of non-cash compensation. The cost of an employer-provided health care plan is essentially passed on to employees through lower cash wages. If employees actually wrote the check for their health insurance premiums, they would be more likely to understand who is really paying for the health care coverage.

Although the preceding discussion about employee compensation appears to have wandered away from the issues of Medicare and Medicaid, it brings up another point. The current generation of workers is effectively paying for four forms of health care:

- Their own health care — through reduced wages or direct premium payments;

- Hospital Insurance for retirees — through payroll taxes to fund Medicare Part A (to be discussed in Chapter 5);

- Supplemental Medical Insurance for retirees — through income taxes to fund a portion of Medicare Part B (to be discussed in Chapter 6);

- Medicaid for the needy — through income taxes (to be discussed in Chapter 8).

The system of having current workers pay for the health care costs of retired workers operated effectively during the early days of the program. One of the primary reasons was that in 1965, there were 4.5 workers for every

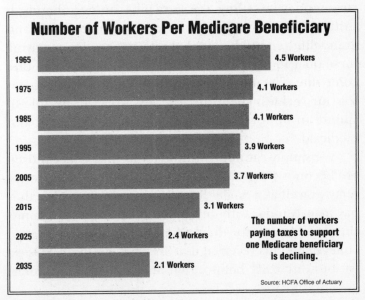

Number of Workers Per Medicare Beneficiary

1965	4.5 Workers
1975	4.1 Workers
1985	4.1 Workers
1995	3.9 Workers
2005	3.7 Workers
2015	3.1 Workers
2025	2.4 Workers
2035	2.1 Workers

The number of workers paying taxes to support one Medicare beneficiary is declining.

Source: HCFA Office of Actuary

retiree. By 1995, there were only 3.9 workers for every retiree. By 2035, there will only be 2.1 workers for every retiree. The graph on page 33 illustrates this declining ratio.

WHO ULTIMATELY PAYS THE BILL?

Who pays for the public health care programs of Medicare and Medicaid? The quick answer is that government pays the bill. The better answer is that taxpayers pay for it. However, the best answer is another question, "Who *ultimately* pays the bill?" The answer to this question leads to the issue of fairness. Is it right to have our children and grandchildren pay our bills?

This is exactly what is happening as a result of our unwillingness to balance the federal budget. We are passing along the cost of our excess spending by borrowing for the things we want today. When the government borrows money by selling Treasury bills, notes or bonds, it shifts the cost to future generations. Our children and grandchildren will be saddled with the burden of paying these obligations of the United States Treasury when they come due. The more that future generations have to pay for our reckless spending, the less they will be able to spend on important programs such as Medicare and Medicaid.

We simply cannot continue to do this. Our children are becoming increasingly cynical about a Medicare system (as well as a Social Security system) for which they pay heavily today with only an empty promise that something will be left for them when they retire. A survey of college students revealed that 46% believe that UFOs exist, but only 28% believe that Social Security will exist when they retire. The reason for their doubt is easy to understand — the debt that continues to grow every year.

Although the college students (or any age group, for that matter) may not have a detailed knowledge of the debt and the deficit, they have an understanding from their everyday experience. They know they cannot spend more than they make without borrowing money from someone. The good news is that most of them understand that they cannot keep borrowing forever. The bad news is that most of them do not yet fully appreciate how difficult it is to repay the principal when they also have to pay interest on the amount borrowed.

The younger generation knows that something is wrong with the current structure of the federal budget — they just don't know exactly what it is. The graph on page 36 illustrates the problem that could be bothering them. Every item in the federal budget is classified as either a *mandatory* expenditure or a *discretionary* expenditure. Mandatory expenditures include Medicare and Medicaid payments, Social Security benefits, other entitlement programs, and interest on the national debt.

Discretionary expenditures can be thought of as any item for which Congress can decide to increase or decrease spending during the budget process. Interestingly, the discretionary category includes expenditures for the national defense, even though a large portion of the military budget might be considered a "fixed" expense. Other discretionary spending items include expenditures for education, highway maintenance, and law enforcement.

- The graph below indicates that in 1964, 70% of government expenditures were for discretionary items, and 30% were for mandatory items.

- By 1994, the ratio had almost reversed itself — 63% of government spending will fall into the mandatory category with only 37% of the budget under the control of Congress.

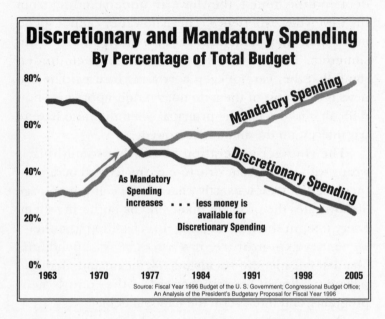

Discretionary and Mandatory Spending
By Percentage of Total Budget

Source: Fiscal Year 1996 Budget of the U. S. Government; Congressional Budget Office; An Analysis of the President's Budgetary Proposal for Fiscal Year 1996

Is it possible that mandatory spending could ever exceed the total amount of revenue that the government collects in taxes and fees? Not only is the answer "Yes," one study has even predicted when it will occur. In 1994, the Kerrey-Danforth Bipartisan Commission on Entitlement and Tax Reform undertook a study to determine, among other things, the impact of entitlement programs, such as Social Security, Medicare, and Medicaid, on the standard of living for this generation and future generations of Americans.

THE BIG PICTURE

The graph on page 38 indicates that if government revenues (mainly taxes) are assumed to average 19% of GDP, as they have for many years now, mandatory spending alone will exceed all tax revenue in the year 2012. If this happens, the government will have to borrow money for every discretionary program that it wants to undertake, including national defense and practically every other typical function of government. For example, the government would have to borrow money every year to operate the national parks, staff the prisons, and even print our money. Of course, by that time, it may be impossible for the United States government to borrow any more money. Our debt level may be so high that investors would be reluctant to buy our Treasury securities.

As noted in the Kerrey-Danforth Commission Report:

> *We acquire a false sense of optimism when we look ahead only five years, as we do with our traditional budgeting process. Only when we look at the next 30 years — the horizon of our children — does the problem and its size come into full view.*

Not only does the five-year budget planning outlook prevent us from grasping the magnitude of the problem, but the procedures for reporting the financial operations of our government would confuse a rocket scientist. It's no wonder. When government officials in Washington talk about a *cut*, they are usually talking about a slower increase in spending than originally projected.

Even worse than confusing us, some of the terms that the government uses in connection with its finances are intentionally misleading. Take the Social Security *trust*

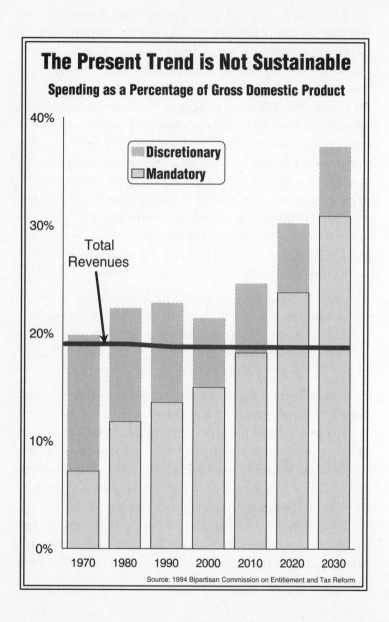

The Present Trend is Not Sustainable

Spending as a Percentage of Gross Domestic Product

Discretionary
Mandatory

Total Revenues

Source: 1994 Bipartisan Commission on Entitlement and Tax Reform

fund and the Medicare *trust fund,* for example. Do these *trust funds* really guarantee that enough money will be available to pay the benefits promised by Medicare and Social Security when the time comes? **DO THESE TRUST FUNDS CONTAIN ANY MONEY?** Chapter 3 will explain what these trust funds contain, and, more importantly, what they don't contain.

LESSONS LEARNED

In 1994, the Clinton Administration proposed a program that would have completely overhauled this nation's entire health care system (including Medicare and Medicaid) and put it under the control of the federal government. Without going into a lengthy post-mortem, two lessons were clear:

- People do not want the government telling them what kind of health care they can and cannot have.

- What is needed is reform of the health care *financing* system that would not jeopardize the quality of health care.

We should learn from past mistakes. The goal of Medicare and Medicaid reform should be to reform their financing systems. A properly designed system based on market principles will do more to bring about positive change than any government rules and regulations which attempt to monitor the profits of the health care industry.

We should view the coming debate over modernizing Medicare and Medicaid as an opportunity rather than a dilemma. It can be an opportunity for creative minds to update old systems that have served their purpose, but are now in need of an overhaul to function properly in the next century. This is an ambitious goal, but the consequences of business-as-usual will only lead to less health care at higher costs for everyone.

3

Beltway Buzzwords

Out of necessity, almost every organization develops terminology and jargon of its own to describe certain unique functions and procedures. Words are given meanings that differ from their everyday definitions. The government of the United States may be the world's leader in this practice. To properly discuss Medicare and Medicaid, it is first necessary to explain how Washington has redefined the term *trust fund* and the word *cut*.

Most people think of a trust fund as a source of money. Universities typically have trust funds that are used to fund special projects or scholarships. The university seeks contributions and places the money in a savings account or secure investment. The money to pay for the special programs is usually taken from the earnings (interest and dividends, for example) of the money that has been placed into the trust funds. By operating in this manner, the original contribution is never touched. It is preserved so that money will be available in the future. This is very prudent, and a sound way of doing business.

INTENSIVE CARE

To receive income from the trust fund, the principal must be invested to earn interest, dividends, or some other form of return on the money. Typically, the cash in these funds is used to purchase interest bearing securities, such as certificates of deposit from banks or the bonds of large corporations.

Some institutions are willing to take more risk to earn a higher return on their principal. In these cases, the trustees of these trust funds might recommend the purchase of stock in companies that are listed on the New York Stock Exchange.

GOVERNMENT TRUST FUNDS

The government of the United States maintains many trust funds — or at least that is what the government calls them. In an attempt to clarify the meaning of a government trust fund, the Congressional Budget Office issued the following definition:

> *A fund, designated as a trust fund by statute, that is credited with income from earmarked collections and charged with certain outlays. Collections may come from the public (for example, taxes or user charges) or from intrabudgetary transfers. More than 150 federal government trust funds exist, of which the largest and best known finance several benefit programs (including Social Security and Medicare) and certain infrastructure spending (the Highway and Airport and Airway Trust Funds).*

If it weren't for the terms *earmarked collections, certain outlays,* and *intrabudgetary transfers,* the above definition might be fairly straightforward. However, it's not a bad start.

BELTWAY BUZZWORDS

To get an idea of how a government trust fund works, imagine that you are a member of a large family. You have a good job, and you are able to pay all of your bills on a timely basis. In fact, you have extra money left over that you would like to save for the future. However, your particular family has an unusual rule about members who have extra money. You, your brothers and sisters, and your cousins are restricted in your ability to invest your money. You cannot put your money into the same types of investments (certificates of deposit, stocks, etc.) that were mentioned above.

You have only one investment option available to you. The head of your extended family is your father's brother — your uncle. His name is Sam. Whenever you have any extra money, you are required to invest your money with Uncle Sam. He promises to pay you back, with interest, whenever you need it. He takes all your money and gives you an IOU. He keeps books, so he makes a notation of how much he owes you.

A year goes by, and you are still doing well. You have more money to invest, so you take it to Uncle Sam. He accepts your money, gives you another IOU, and makes another entry in his books. As you are driving home, you ask yourself, "Will Uncle Sam be able to repay the money that I am investing with him? **WHAT IS UNCLE SAM DOING WITH ALL THIS MONEY?**"

We could repeat this story year after year into your retirement years, but let's return to government trust funds. A government trust fund is similar to your situation in the above example. The trust fund takes in money (from payroll taxes, for example) and makes payments for specified items (to Medicare beneficiaries, for example). If there is any money left over, the trustees of the trust fund are required to invest the money with the federal government by purchasing Treasury bills, bonds, or notes from the United States government. They have no choice in the matter about what to do with the extra money — they *must* purchase U.S. Treasury securities.

When the securities mature, the federal government owes the money, plus the accumulated interest, to the trust funds. However, the government is not required to maintain a pool of money to repay this obligation. Instead, it adds the money that it receives from the trust funds to the other money that it gets directly from income taxes and other sources. The government then spends all of this money each year. In effect, any excess money that is supposed to go into the Medicare trust fund, for example, is being spent on everything from agriculture subsidies to zoos.

As noted in Chapter 2, to make up the difference between money spent and money received, the government borrows money from outside sources — from non-family members, so to speak. The amount borrowed each year from outside sources is defined as the deficit for the year.

The chart on page 45 indicates the largest trust funds to which the federal government owes money. In accounting terms, the amount of money that the federal government owes to a trust fund is a *liability* of the federal government. In plain talk, the taxpayers have to pay the money some day. On the other side of the ledger, the amount of money owed to a trust fund is considered to be an *asset* of that trust fund.

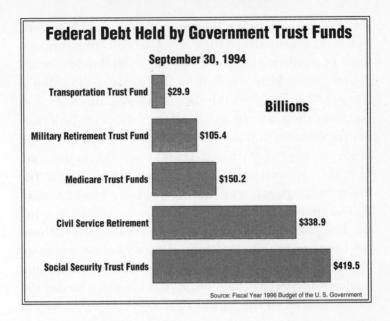

Federal Debt Held by Government Trust Funds

September 30, 1994

Transportation Trust Fund — $29.9

Billions

Military Retirement Trust Fund — $105.4

Medicare Trust Funds — $150.2

Civil Service Retirement — $338.9

Social Security Trust Funds — $419.5

Source: Fiscal Year 1996 Budget of the U. S. Government

The table below shows the composition of the federal debt at the end of the latest fiscal year, September 30, 1994.

National Debt September 30, 1994	
Debt held by the public	$3,432,213,000,000
Debt held by gov't trust funds	$1,211,498,000,000
Total National Debt	**$4,643,711,000,000**

In everyday terms, the above discussion results in this situation: assume that you were allowed to walk into the offices of the Health Care Financing Administration

(HCFA) and ask to see the assets of the Medicare Trust Fund. The only thing they *might* be able to show you would be pieces of paper from the federal government representing $150.2 billion in IOUs. More than likely, you would be shown a number on a computer screen. If you were then able to walk into the offices of the Treasury Department and ask where they were going to get the money to pay the Medicare Trust Fund, they would have to reply, "We will get it from the taxpayers." These are the same taxpayers who already paid the $150.2 billion that was borrowed from the trust fund.

The point of this discussion is that there is no money held in reserve that can be used to pay excess Medicare claims. Interest is rolled forward and compounded, dramatically increasing the burden to taxpayers. The day will soon come when the Medicare trust fund begins paying out more money in claims than it receives in payroll taxes. In fact, the chart below indicates that it will occur in 1996.

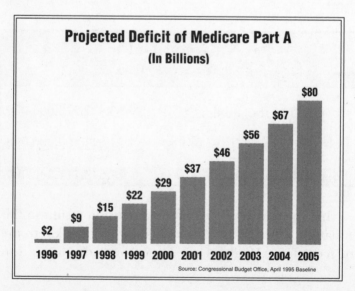

Projected Deficit of Medicare Part A
(In Billions)

1996	1997	1998	1999	2000	2001	2002	2003	2004	2005
$2	$9	$15	$22	$29	$37	$46	$56	$67	$80

Source: Congressional Budget Office, April 1995 Baseline

The Ways and Means Committee of the House of Representatives has described this situation clearly, "When the trust funds' IOUs are needed...the Government will have to raise taxes, curtail other expenditures, or increase its borrowing from the public."

It seems contradictory for the federal government to require companies to keep their pension funds adequately funded. The government should impose the same requirement on itself.

THE DEBT AND THE DEFICIT . . . AGAIN

It seems that all roads lead back to the debt and the deficit, and the trust fund discussion is no exception.

The trust funds play a misleading and confusing role in the calculation of the debt and the deficit. This can best be explained with an example.

At the beginning of the government's 1994 fiscal year, the national debt was calculated to be approximately $4.3 trillion. By the end of the year, the debt was approximately $4.6 trillion. More precise numbers are shown below.

Change in the National Debt	
September 30, 1994	$4.643 trillion
September 30, 1993	$4.351 trillion
Increase in National Debt	**$0.292 trillion**

The increase in the national debt was $292 billion for the fiscal year ending September 30, 1994. However, the table below indicates that the government reported a deficit of only $203 billion — the amount that it borrowed from the public during the year.

So What's the Difference?	
Increase in National Debt	$292 billion
Deficit for the year	$203 billion
Difference	**$ 89 billion**

SO, WHY IS THERE AN $89 BILLION DIFFERENCE?

The answer is that the government trust funds lent the federal government $89 billion during 1994, but the government does not report that amount as part of *the deficit.* On the other hand, when the government reports the total amount of the national debt, it includes the amount that is owed to the trust funds in its calculation of *the debt.*

The reason for the inconsistent reporting treatment of the deficit and the debt dates back to President Johnson's attempt to handle the escalating budget deficits during the Vietnam War. This practice continues today as the reported amount of the annual budget deficit does not include the amount of money that had to be borrowed from the various trust funds to operate the government during the year.

REGARDLESS OF WHAT WASHINGTON REPORTS THE DEFICIT TO BE, THE DIFFERENCE BETWEEN GOVERNMENT INCOME AND SPENDING IS HOW MUCH THE DEBT RISES FROM ONE YEAR TO THE NEXT.

BELTWAY BUZZWORDS

THE UNKINDEST CUT OF ALL

The budget is also involved in another misleading government practice. This misdirection will be on display throughout the Medicare and Medicaid debate. It concerns the use of the word *cut* in connection with the budget.

Despite all of the talk about cutting this program or that program, we still have a budget deficit and the debt continues to increase. The problem begins with a requirement that the President's annual budget include a five-year projection for spending. These projections always indicate that government spending will increase.

The graph on page 50 shows three levels of spending. The upper line represents the projected increases in spending for Medicare under the Clinton Administration's original budget proposed for fiscal year 1996. Those figures indicate an average rate of increase of 10.1% from 1995 through the year 2000.

The lower line serves as a reference to indicate the actual level of Medicare spending in 1995. In other words, if Medicare costs did not increase or decrease after 1995, the government would continue to spend $178 billion on Medicare each year.

The line in the middle indicates the level of spending proposed for Medicare in the House budget plan that was passed on May 18, 1995. The House proposal would attempt to hold Medicare spending increases to 5.89% per year. This reduces the rate of growth of Medicare. Only in Washington would this be called a spending cut.

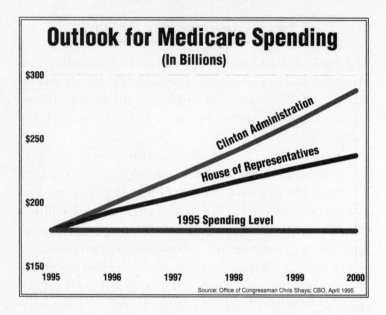

Outlook for Medicare Spending
(In Billions)

Source: Office of Congressman Chris Shays; CBO, April 1995

The House proposal has been attacked and will continue to be attacked as a spending cut in the Medicare program. When the term "spending cut" is applied to a situation such as this, it is used for no other reason than to deceive innocent taxpayers into believing that someone is trying to reduce the amount of their benefits. It is deception at its worst.

In a reasoned explanation two years earlier, President Clinton made the statement shown below.

> *Today, Medicaid and Medicare are going up at three times the rate of inflation. We propose to let it go up at two times the rate of inflation. That is not a Medicare or Medicaid cut. So when you hear all this business about cuts, let me caution you that that is not what is going on. We are going to have increases in Medicare and Medicaid, and a reduction in the rate of growth.*

BELTWAY BUZZWORDS

Both the President and Congress agree that Medicare spending and Medicaid spending need to be controlled. There is widespread agreement that Medicare and Medicaid spending is not being cut. The next step is to put political jargon aside and work together to modernize Medicare and Medicaid.

4

Medicare:
A Growth Industry

All of the accounting gimmicks and political jargon that Washington devises cannot hide one fact: the cost of Medicare is growing too fast. Lawmakers have known about the poor financial condition of Medicare for years. Instead of reforming the system and improving the long-term future of Medicare, the legislative surgeons in Congress have applied Band-Aids where major surgery was needed. Outside of Congress this negligence would be called malpractice. Inside Congress it is called politics.

Medicare spending will double every five to seven years under current conditions. A trend of this magnitude cannot be sustained for long. The chart on page 54 shows how fast Medicare spending is expected to increase. Between 1995 and 2003 Medicare spending will more than double.

As Medicare spending rises higher and higher, the chance of ever balancing the federal budget becomes less

likely. Modernizing Medicare and improving its long-term financial prospects is necessary to save the system for *every* American.

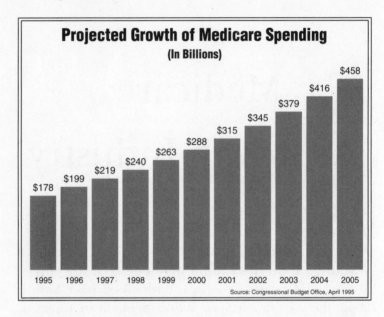

Projected Growth of Medicare Spending
(In Billions)

1995	$178
1996	$199
1997	$219
1998	$240
1999	$263
2000	$288
2001	$315
2002	$345
2003	$379
2004	$416
2005	$458

Source: Congressional Budget Office, April 1995

The primary threat to Medicare is rising costs. Controlling the growth of Medicare costs is the yardstick that must be used to measure every reform proposal. If a reform measure cannot control rising costs, then what is the point of reforming the current system?

OVER THE PAST 20 YEARS THE COST OF THE ENTIRE MEDICARE PROGRAM HAS INCREASED AN AVERAGE OF ALMOST 15% A YEAR. This extraordinary growth rate caused the percentage of total federal spending required by just Medicare to more than triple during the 20-year period. In 1974 the program was responsible for 3.4% of all federal spending. By 1995 Medicare alone will account for 11.6% of all federal spending.

MEDICARE: A GROWTH INDUSTRY

The growth rate of Medicare will only continue to rise if no real reforms are adopted. As the chart below indicates, Medicare is expected to consume increasing portions of the federal budget during the next decade. **IN JUST TEN YEARS, BY THE YEAR 2005, MEDICARE IS EXPECTED TO ABSORB 18.5% OF ALL FEDERAL SPENDING.**

These projections, of course, are from the federal government. It is unlikely that these estimates will be as inaccurate as the earlier numbers shown on page 7, but this does not necessarily mean that the projections are flawless.

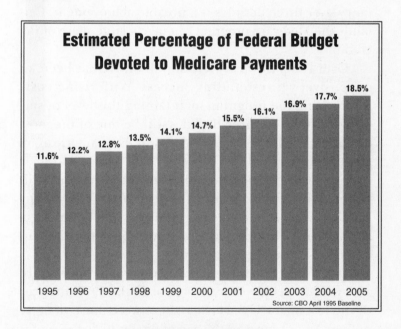

AN AGING SOCIETY

Rising costs in Medicare cannot be blamed on a single culprit. There are many different factors contributing to the problem. Many more factors probably have not yet been discovered. Determining and defining Medicare's ills is essential to real and lasting reform. A doctor must diagnose what is wrong with a patient before a treatment is prescribed.

Certainly, the growing number of senior citizens in America is contributing to the increasing costs experienced by the Medicare system. Longer life spans also contribute to increased health care requirements.

In 1965 a person who was 65 years old could expect to live another 14.5 years. By 1995 this figure had increased to 17.5 years. A three-year increase in life expectancy over three decades is a notable achievement. Certainly the Medicare program can take a large share of the credit.

Over the past three decades Medicare has been an expensive, yet resounding success. With rising costs threatening the program, maintaining this level of success over the *next* three decades will be one of the most important challenges our leaders will face. American ingenuity must prevail.

The largest generation of Americans ever born will begin retiring shortly after the year 2010. These Baby Boomers will begin collecting Medicare and Social Security benefits. This will place an enormous financial burden on the federal government.

In 1965, the year Medicare was created, there were 18.5 million people over the age of 65. By 1990, the year of the last major U.S. census, there were more than 31 million Americans over the age of 65. By 2020, the senior citizen population is expected to increase to 54 million people. **DURING THE 30-YEAR PERIOD FROM 1990 TO 2020, THE GROWTH RATE OF THE SENIOR CITIZEN POPULATION**

MEDICARE: A GROWTH INDUSTRY

WILL BE DOUBLE THE GROWTH RATE OF THE TOTAL U.S. POPULATION.

What does all this mean? As shown on page 33, the retired population that collects entitlement benefits such as Social Security and Medicare will grow faster than the working population that pays taxes. In business terms, costs will grow faster than revenues.

One of the fastest growing and most expensive age groups will be the senior citizens who live past the age of 85. The average 85-year-old Medicare recipient is twice as expensive to care for as the average 65-year-old recipient.

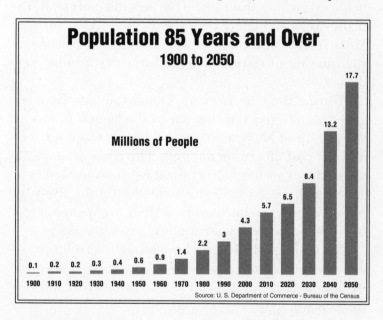

Population 85 Years and Over
1900 to 2050

Millions of People

1900	1910	1920	1930	1940	1950	1960	1970	1980	1990	2000	2010	2020	2030	2040	2050
0.1	0.2	0.2	0.3	0.4	0.6	0.9	1.4	2.2	3	4.3	5.7	6.5	8.4	13.2	17.7

Source: U. S. Department of Commerce - Bureau of the Census

As the chart above indicates, the 85-and-over age group is growing rapidly. By 2050, there are expected to be 17.7 million people over 85 years old. This will be an increase of almost 600% from the 85-and-over population in 1990.

INTENSIVE CARE

Common sense dictates that the older a person gets, the more health care he or she needs. An 80-year-old should require more health care than a 60-year-old, and a 60-year-old should require more health care than a 40-year-old. This is simply a fact of life. So once again we return to a common denominator — the need to control rising costs.

AN EXPENSIVE SOCIETY

Americans are living longer because technology has made everything from a heart bypass to an organ transplant easier and safer. Technology, like CAT scans and MRIs, has also increased health care costs and increased the number of tests and procedures that can be conducted.

During the next 15 years, before the Baby Boomer generation begins retiring, one of the biggest factors in the growth of Medicare costs will be increased services and the cost of new technology. The chart on page 59 shows the expected sources for the growth in Medicare spending between 1995 and 1999. Within this five-year period almost two-thirds of new Medicare spending will be a result of increased services and new technology.

Technological advances have brought health care — as well as health care costs — to new heights. As the quality of health care has increased, so has its cost and the frequency of its use.

When the Medicare program was created 30 years ago, lasers were thought of as dangerous weapons straight from science fiction movies. Today, lasers are used routinely as surgical tools. Laser surgery is not inexpensive.

MEDICARE: A GROWTH INDUSTRY

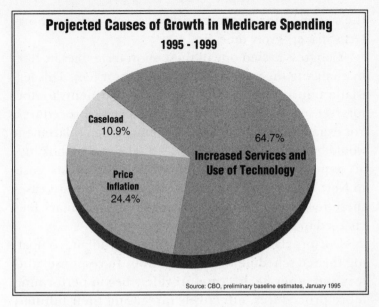

Projected Causes of Growth in Medicare Spending
1995 - 1999

Caseload
10.9%

64.7%
Increased Services and
Use of Technology

Price
Inflation
24.4%

Source: CBO, preliminary baseline estimates, January 1995

Thirty years ago the only medical alternative for a heart patient was open heart surgery. Today, doctors use miniature camera lenses on tiny catheters that only require a small incision to look inside a patient's heart. Blocked arteries can be cleared using similar catheters. Heart attacks can now be more easily prevented. As a result, deaths by heart disease are declining. Heart procedures are not inexpensive either.

Today's patients are experiencing better care. Better care often means more care, and more care usually means more money. Medicare, which was designed 30 years ago, must be modernized to deal with this situation.

Medicare spending seems to increase as rapidly as advances in technology. **THE PROBLEM IS THE TAX BASE THAT FINANCES MEDICARE IS NOT KEEPING PACE.**

Congress has attempted to control costs in the past with weak reforms that have not changed the nature of the system. Short-term repairs have won out over long-term answers every time.

Congress passed one of these short-term fixes in 1989 by changing the way Medicare pays doctor fees. This legislation introduced a fee schedule for payments to doctors, setting predetermined fees for specific procedures. For example, every doctor performing a hip replacement would be paid a predetermined fee. The system took into account geographical differences in medical costs; costs in New York are higher than in Montana. In most cases these fees were less than the usual and customary fees charged by health care providers.

Doctors claimed these payments were unfair, comparing the fee schedule to price controls. In response, doctors and other health care providers began performing more procedures, effectively increasing their billings. This practice of using more procedures and tests is known as "intensity" which has been a large contributor to Medicare's rising costs. This practice is legal as long as the procedures are actually performed and are deemed necessary.

The government's plan has backfired. Doctors found a way to make up for their losses.

OUR POLITICAL LEADERS MUST LEARN THAT ARTIFICIALLY HOLDING DOWN PAYMENTS IS NOT A SUBSTITUTE FOR MEANINGFUL REFORM.

AN EXPENSIVE SYSTEM

One of the largest contributors to the rising cost of Medicare is the method that is used to pay health care providers. The current Medicare system is basically a fee-for-service arrangement. Hospitals, doctors and other providers are paid a majority of a beneficiary's bill directly from Medicare for each test and procedure performed. On average, Medicare beneficiaries only pay about 16% of the cost from their own pocket. The problem is that fee-for-service medicine offers few incentives for doctors or patients to use health care in a cost-effective manner.

For doctors, Medicare started out as a fair deal. They treated Medicare patients and the government paid the bill, but times have changed. Today, doctors are paid according to the restrictive Medicare fee schedule that was previously mentioned.

Most doctors, whether in private practice or employed by someone else, are part of a business whose goal is to cover its costs and earn a profit. This is not to imply that compensation is their primary goal in life. It just recognizes the fact that the continuing practice of medicine requires some financial success. To improve profits a business must either cut costs or raise prices. In medicine costs are difficult to cut, so raising prices is the only alternative.

Because of the capped Medicare fee schedule, doctors cannot raise prices. The only other way to increase revenue is to perform more tests and procedures that may only be marginally necessary. As a result, the government and patients have a larger health care bill to pay.

Fee-for-service medicine has also caused many Medicare recipients to take advantage of the system. Because Medicare pays for a majority of a beneficiary's health care costs, beneficiaries have little incentive to reduce their use of the health care system and save money.

WHEN MEDICARE RECIPIENTS GO TO A DOCTOR, THEY RARELY ASK, "HOW MUCH IS THIS GOING TO COST?"

If the government is paying the largest portion of the health care bill, many people do not worry about the price. The current fee-for-service system used by most Medicare recipients does not encourage patients to inquire about fees. A variety of reform alternatives that address this problem will be discussed in Chapter 7.

AN ABUSED SYSTEM

Waste, fraud and abuse in the Medicare system are costing American taxpayers billions of dollars every year. Cheating the Medicare system has become a multi-billion dollar industry in the United States. Because the system is so complex and growing so fast, it has been an easy target for crooks and cheats.

In the early 1980s one Medicare fraud scheme in California is estimated to have collected $1 *billion* in fraudulent claims. This operation relied on "rolling labs," which were vans carrying portable medical equipment. The portable laboratories would visit nursing homes, health clubs, and churches to attract patients.

The operators would often give false and misleading information about certain diseases to attract customers. They would tell people that the portable lab could conduct the appropriate tests. Telemarketing was even used to contact potential customers at home.

The patients were attracted to the program because they were not required to pay a cent out of their own pocket. Instead, the company would bill Medicare or private insurance companies for tests that were not necessary or sometimes were not even performed.

Even though these rolling labs were widespread, state and federal officials did not have the technology and safeguards to detect the fraud. Over a 10-year period the labs operated under at least 500 different names with hundreds of physicians involved.

This is not a unique story in the business of Medicare fraud. It just illustrates how Medicare is out of control and how few safeguards are in place.

In 1983 a U.S. General Accounting Office study found even more fraud associated with this vast operation. **ONE DOCTOR'S MEDICARE BILLINGS INCREASED FROM $18,953 TO $188,241 OVER A THREE-MONTH PERIOD!**

It was also revealed that the owners of the rolling labs were paying kickbacks to doctors for referring patients to the labs. Under this arrangement, the lab operators would pay doctors a set fee for each patient who was referred to the labs.

In 1986 one of the owners of the rolling labs was arrested, but the labs continued to operate. Instead of taking advantage of senior citizens, the labs focused on health clubs and began testing people with private insurance. As late as 1991 indictments were still being handed down in connection with the Medicare swindle.

Medicare fraud is still alive and well today. Many past offenders come back to defraud the government. In May 1995 one of the country's largest medical testing laboratories agreed to pay $8.6 million to settle allegations that the company had defrauded the federal government. Only two years earlier the company had agreed to a $35 million settlement with the government on claims for unnecessary blood tests. The company denied any wrongdoing in both cases.

During a two-year period this company has paid $43.6 million to settle fraud allegations. In the private sector a business would stop using a contractor who is supposedly using questionable billing practices. The government, on the other hand, continues to use this company as a Medicare provider.

While Medicare and the company continue this love/hate relationship, there is a bright side to this story. A former employee originally sued the company claiming that it routinely charged Medicare for tests that were never performed. She sued under a *whistle-blower* law passed during the Civil War that allows citizens to sue a company if the government is being defrauded. The Justice Department then intervened in the case.

The former employee made it her personal responsibility to stop fraud against the United States government. As a result she will receive $1.29 million of the latest settlement with the company.

To help detect and combat waste, fraud and abuse Medicare is now designing new systems that will uncover signs of fraud and abuse. When Medicare claims from a health care provider increase at an unusual pace, the new system will alert Medicare officials. How well this system will work remains to be seen. It is at least three years away from completion.

New systems will be helpful, but they will never replace concerned Americans who report fraud in the health care system. **MEDICARE BENEFICIARIES SHOULD BE REWARDED FOR REPORTING FRAUD TO THE GOVERNMENT. IF EVERY MEDICARE BENEFICIARY HAD THE MOTIVATION TO SCRUTINIZE THEIR BILLS AND TO REPORT INSTANCES OF FRAUD AND ABUSE, WE WOULD HAVE 36 MILLION INSPECTORS THROUGHOUT THE SYSTEM.**

MEDICARE: A GROWTH INDUSTRY

DOUBLE TROUBLE

Medicare's costs are out of control for various reasons. The larger the program becomes and the more people it covers, the more difficult it is to oversee. When a program is allowed to grow at an unmanageable pace, its collapse is almost inevitable.

The entire Medicare problem becomes more complex because Medicare is actually two separate programs covering 36 million people. The first program is the Hospital Insurance portion known as *Medicare Part A*. The second program is the Supplemental Medical Insurance portion known as *Medicare Part B*.

Part A pays for hospital services, and Part B pays for doctors' services. Most of the 36 million Medicare beneficiaries are enrolled in both programs.

Part A and Part B are intended to complement each other. If a beneficiary needs surgery, Part A would help pay the hospital costs while Part B would help pay the surgeon's bill. Both programs have the same goal of providing quality health care, and both programs are suffering from many of the same problems.

When reform proposals are discussed, the possibility of combining Medicare Part A and B should be on the agenda. Hospitals and most doctors cannot survive without each other. So why should the programs that pay them be separate?

Chapters 5 and 6 will discuss Medicare Part A and Part B in more detail. First, we need to take a look at the eligibility, financing, and coverage under these two programs that 36 million people rely on for their health care needs.

INTENSIVE CARE

ELIGIBILITY

You are automatically eligible for Medicare Part A if you fall under at least one of the following categories:

- You are at least 65 years old and eligible for Social Security benefits or you are receiving railroad retirement. Almost 90% of all Medicare Part A recipients fall under this category.
- If you are at least 65 years old but are not eligible for or receiving either of the benefits above, you can receive benefits by paying a monthly premium, which is $261 in 1995.
- You are disabled and have been receiving Social Security or railroad retirement disability benefits for 24 months.
- You are diagnosed with end stage renal disease (kidney failure) and you meet certain eligibility requirements.

The requirements for Medicare Part B are much more simple than for Part A. This program is open to:

- Anyone enrolled in Medicare Part A who pays the monthly premium, which is $46.10 in 1995.
- Anyone not enrolled in Medicare Part A, but who is at least 65 years old, can join Medicare Part B for the same monthly premium.

FINANCING

As you will learn in the next two chapters, the financing for Medicare Part A and B are completely separate. Medicare Part A is almost exclusively financed by a payroll tax collected from everyone who is employed or self-employed in the United States. Revenue for Medicare Part A is generated from:

MEDICARE: A GROWTH INDUSTRY

- A 1.45% payroll tax on the wages of all employees and an equal 1.45% tax on employers.
- A 2.9% payroll tax on the earnings of the self-employed.
- Premiums paid by enrollees who are over 65 but do not qualify for Social Security or railroad retirement benefits.
- Interest from the Part A trust fund.

Medicare Part B is financed through income taxes paid by hard working men and women. Revenue for Medicare Part B is generated from:

- Monthly premiums of $46.10 for 1995.
- General revenue from the U.S. Treasury

COVERAGE

Medicare Part A covers the costs associated with hospital care that include:

- Inpatient hospital care
- Short term skilled nursing facility care
- Home health care
- Hospice care

Medicare Part B covers the costs related to services that include:

- Doctors' services
- Diagnostic and lab tests, such as X-rays
- Outpatient hospital services
- Physical and speech therapy
- Home dialysis supplies and equipment
- Ambulance services

In addition to the above information related to coverage, Appendices A and B at the back of this book contain a history of the Medicare program. These summaries explain the various forms of coverage that Congress has added to Medicare throughout the history of the program.

Medicare Part A and Medicare Part B do not pick up the entire tab for health care. Part A, for example, requires beneficiaries to pay the first $716 of each hospital stay of 60 days or less. Part B requires a $100 annual deductible, which means that you must pay for the first $100 of your medical care each year. Also, Part B only pays for 80% of most doctors' services. Neither Medicare program covers prescription drugs, eyeglasses, or dental care. The details of Medicare Part A and Medicare Part B will be discussed in greater detail in Chapters 5 and 6, respectively.

Because Medicare does not cover all medical costs, many insurance companies offer supplemental policies, known as *Medigap* insurance. Approximately 75% of Medicare beneficiaries are also covered by Medigap policies or similar supplemental insurance.

In the past, Medigap policies were often ineffective and often associated with fraud and abuse. To combat fraud, the federal government has developed 10 different standard Medigap packages that private insurance companies can sell. Each plan contains the same basic set of benefits.

In addition to these plans, the federal government has also placed restrictions on so-called *pre-existing condition* exclusions. These restrictions prevent insurance companies from denying coverage or canceling an existing policy on individuals with a known physical problem or disease.

The combination of Medicare Part A, Part B, and Medigap policies has not resulted in lower costs to Medicare recipients. The chart below indicates that Medicare beneficiaries are spending more of their own money.

Over the past 20 years out-of-pocket costs for Medicare recipients have increased about 10% a year. Any real reform proposal must also address this issue. Health care costs for the government *and* Medicare beneficiaries are both growing too fast.

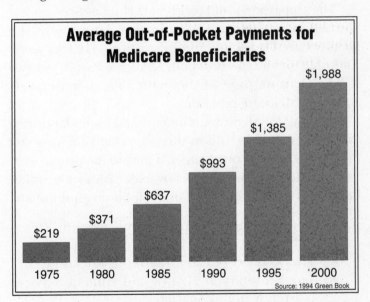

Average Out-of-Pocket Payments for Medicare Beneficiaries

1975	1980	1985	1990	1995	2000
$219	$371	$637	$993	$1,385	$1,988

Source: 1994 Green Book

WHO IS IN CONTROL?

Medicare is an enormous program. Thirty-six million people — more than the entire population of California

— depend on it for their health care. The price tag is $178 billion a year and growing. It involves two separate programs. It must monitor and police beneficiaries, doctors, hospitals, other health care providers, and insurance companies. So, who oversees this enormous program?

Medicare was formed in 1965 through amendments to the Social Security Act. The words *Social Security Act* are even printed on Medicare cards. Financing for Medicare Part A comes from a portion of the Social Security payroll tax deductions. However, in typical government fashion, Medicare is *not* run by the Social Security Administration.

The Department of Health and Human Services has control over Medicare. Within this department the Health Care Financing Administration (HCFA) is responsible for all aspects of both Medicare Part A and Part B. The chart on page 71 shows the bureaucratic layers above the Medicare program.

Funding for Medicare is determined each year during the budget process. It is at this time that Congress and the President settle on changes, if any, to the program.

The Medicare program is overseen by a six-member Board of Trustees composed of the following individuals:

- The Secretary of the Treasury (currently Robert Rubin)
- The Secretary of Labor (currently Robert Reich)
- The Secretary of Health and Human Services (currently Donna Shalala)
- The Commissioner of Social Security (currently Shirley Chater)
- Two public members

MEDICARE: A GROWTH INDUSTRY

Traditionally, one public member is a Democrat and the other a Republican. One of these members is usually nominated by the President, and the other public member is usually nominated by the Senate leader of the opposition party. Once confirmed by the Senate both public Trustees serve four-year terms.

Every year the financial status of Medicare is reported to Congress and the President by the Board of Trustees. The Board delivers two reports, one on the Hospital Insurance Trust Fund (Part A) and the other on the Supplemental Medical Insurance Trust Fund (Part B).

Medicare and the Federal Bureaucracy

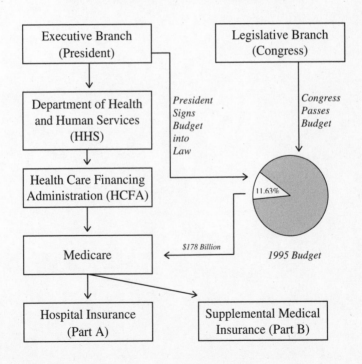

INTENSIVE CARE

Since the early 1970s the Trustees have been warning that the long-term financial condition of Medicare was extremely poor. Every year Congress and the White House, for the most part, ignore the warnings. Minor reforms were passed, but major changes were avoided.

Suddenly, when the 1995 Medicare Board of Trustees report was released, the news of Medicare's pending collapse became the hot topic in Washington. **SOMEONE FINALLY NOTICED THE WARNING LIGHTS THAT HAD BEEN FLASHING FOR TWO DECADES.**

5

Medicare Part A: Bankrupt in 2002

Our airplane has lost a considerable amount of altitude since this flight began. The crew has been watching the instruments and making adjustments, but the plane has fallen to a dangerously low level. Some of the corrections are working because the rate of descent has slowed somewhat. However, nothing seems to be working to make the plane climb.

One of the extra navigators in the expanded cockpit has been curious about a particular warning light since the flight began. The light has become covered with dust and dirt to the point that it cannot be read. He taps on the instrument panel to knock away some of the dust, and suddenly the light begins to flash brightly. He rubs away the dirt, and the label reads MEDICARE PART A.

The navigator immediately notifies the other members of the flight crew. The crew members begin to react in a knowing manner as if it were some secret they had been keeping. "Medicare Part A is failing and needs to be repaired," they begin to tell one another confidently.

For some reason, the report of the Medicare Board of Trustees seems to have gotten a similar reaction in Congress in 1995. The warning lights of the report have been flashing for years, but no one noticed until now. Congress and the President are now talking about Medicare Part A.

The Hospital Insurance Trust Fund, Medicare Part A, will be bankrupt within the next ten years. Under current conditions the fund will technically run out of money in the year 2002 or sooner.

Beginning as soon as 1996, the payroll taxes paid by current workers will not be sufficient to pay the Medicare benefits for current beneficiaries. The shortfall is supposed to be made up from the trust fund. Since the trust fund doesn't have any real money, the government will have to raise taxes or borrow more money. Even if there were money in the trust fund, it would be depleted in only seven years.

The technical issue of the Medicare Part A trust fund going bankrupt will force Congress to deal with the problem. If the program is not updated, then Congress will have to find a way to make the trust fund financially sound. The following options are available to Congress:

- Increasing payroll taxes

- Reducing the rate of growth for spending on Medicare Part A

- A combination of the above

None of these choices is politically popular. With a national crisis quickly approaching, Congress will be forced to act. A fundamental change, not a political quick-fix, is desperately needed.

The financial status report for Medicare Part A came directly from the members of the Board of Trustees for the Hospital Insurance Trust Fund. As the guardians of the trust fund, the Trustees warned that danger is on its way. In their 1995 report, the Trustees said:

> *The HI (Hospital Insurance) program is severely out of financial balance and the Trustees believe that the Congress must take timely action to establish long-term financial stability for the program....The Trustees believe that prompt, effective, and decisive action is necessary.*

IN PLAIN TALK, MEDICARE PART A IS GOING BANKRUPT AND SOMETHING MUST BE DONE IMMEDIATELY TO SAVE THE PROGRAM.

THE ROAD TO BANKRUPTCY

For 20 out of the 30 years it has been in operation, Medicare Part A has received more income than it paid out for health care claims. Every year that it had a surplus, the extra money was placed into the Hospital Insurance Trust Fund. By the end of 1995 this account should be worth approximately $136 billion.

As the chart on page 76 indicates, beginning next year Medicare Part A costs will exceed revenues. This means the program will be running a budget deficit. To cover its deficit Medicare will have to withdraw money from its savings account, the Hospital Insurance Trust Fund. According to the Congressional Budget Office, by the year 2002 Medicare Part A will need to withdraw $160 billion from the trust fund to cover its expenses.

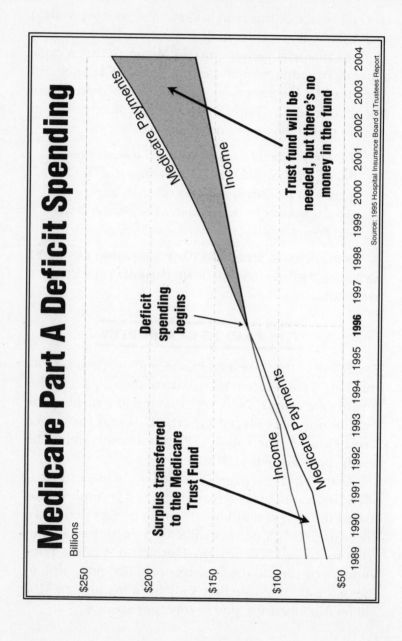

Medicare Part A Deficit Spending

Billions

Medicare Payments

Income

**Surplus transferred
to the Medicare
Trust Fund**

**Deficit
spending
begins**

Income

Medicare Payments

**Trust fund will be
needed, but there's no
money in the fund**

$250

$200

$150

$100

$50

1989 1990 1991 1992 1993 1994 1995 **1996** 1997 1998 1999 2000 2001 2002 2003 2004

Source: 1995 Hospital Insurance Board of Trustees Report

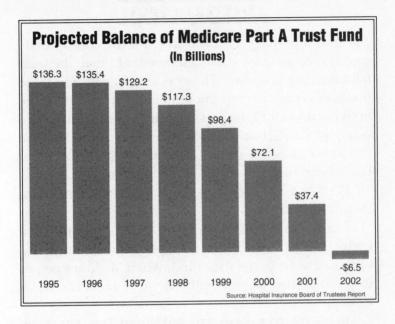

Projected Balance of Medicare Part A Trust Fund
(In Billions)

$136.3 — 1995
$135.4 — 1996
$129.2 — 1997
$117.3 — 1998
$98.4 — 1999
$72.1 — 2000
$37.4 — 2001
-$6.5 — 2002

Source: Hospital Insurance Board of Trustees Report

The problem is the Hospital Insurance Trust Fund will only have $136 billion theoretically available. The facts are this $136 billion already has been spent for something other than Medicare benefits. **TAXPAYERS WILL HAVE TO PAY ADDITIONAL TAXES TO MAKE UP FOR THE MISSING MONEY AS IT IS NEEDED.** The chart above reveals how quickly all the money that is owed to the trust fund by the government will be spent. It has taken 31 years to build up the fund. It will take only 6 years to spend all the savings, which we know has already been spent on other government programs. This is a textbook example of denial and neglect on the part of our elected government officials. The Trustees gave Congress early and sufficient warnings. **CONGRESS IGNORED THE WARNINGS AND CONTINUED TO SPEND THE MEDICARE SAVINGS.**

INTENSIVE CARE

A MATTER OF TRUST

The graph on page 76 illustrates how the cost of Medicare Part A will grow at a much faster pace than the taxes paid into the program. The gray area in between these two lines represents the amount of money that Medicare must borrow. Until the year 2002, this money would have come from the Hospital Insurance Trust Fund. Because this money has been spent, Medicare will be forced to borrow even more money from the taxpayers.

EITHER WAY THE MONEY MUST ULTIMATELY COME FROM THE TAXPAYERS.

Starting in 1996 Medicare Part A will begin running a budget deficit, and will need to spend the money that is supposed to be in the trust fund. When Medicare begins to use this trust fund, it will have to redeem the IOUs from the U.S. Treasury.

IN ORDER TO PAY OFF THE IOUs, THE U.S. TREASURY WILL HAVE TO USE MONEY FROM THE FEDERAL GOVERNMENT'S GENERAL REVENUES.

The federal government, however, does not have extra money to give away. It is already spending about $200 billion a year more than it can afford. When the time comes to pay back the Hospital Insurance Trust Fund, the government will be forced to borrow even more money. As a result, the national debt will rise even higher. **A LARGER DEBT WILL RESULT IN LARGER INTEREST PAYMENTS. LARGER INTEREST PAYMENTS WILL RESULT IN LESS MONEY BEING AVAILABLE FOR PROGRAMS SUCH AS MEDICARE.**

MEDICARE PART A: BANKRUPT IN 2002

OLD NEWS

As far back as 1978 the Medicare Board of Trustees warned that the Hospital Insurance Trust Fund was going bankrupt. Back then they said it would happen in 1990.

With a tax increase and a few patchwork reforms, Congress delayed the technical bankruptcy of Medicare Part A for a few more years. Once again a temporary solution was found while a long term, permanent answer was avoided.

The 1991 Trustees' report revealed that the financial condition of Medicare Part A had temporarily improved. At that time the trust fund was expected to survive until the year 2005 if conditions remained the same. The year 2005 was 14 years away enabling Congress and the White House to ignore the Medicare problem for a few more years.

The 1991 Medicare Trustees' report also noted that if conditions affecting health care deteriorated, the trust fund was likely to be bankrupt in the year 2001. The nation's leaders chose to ignore that warning because 2005 was further away and therefore the problem did not seem as immediate.

The 1995 Trustees' report predicts Medicare Part A will be bankrupt in 2002, making the 2001 projection more accurate than the 2005 projection. Conditions affecting health care costs obviously have worsened since 1991.

The Trustees' 1995 prediction that Medicare Part A will go bankrupt in 2002 was made under the assumption that health care conditions would remain the same from 1995 through 2002. If conditions get worse, they project that the program may be bankrupt a year earlier, in 2001.

INTENSIVE CARE

TAXING AND SPENDING

Over the years, Washington's prescription for troubled federal programs has been to spend more money on them. The money for increased spending was obtained either through higher taxes or borrowing, which delays the need for new taxes until the debt is due.

Medicare's uncontrolled need for money has been treated with higher taxes and reduced payments to health care providers. Eighty-seven percent of the income for Medicare Part A comes from the payroll tax. Congress has always found it easier to increase the payroll tax than to modernize the 30-year-old system and control its outrageous growth. Increasing taxes is always an easier answer than solving the problem.

This is how the Medicare Part A payroll tax works for employees and self-employed individuals. Assume that a self-employed individual, who previously had no employees, hired a recent college graduate at a salary of $24,000.00 per year. The employee will be paid twice a month. Therefore, his or her salary before any withholding is $1,000.00 per paycheck.

Because the Medicare tax rate is 1.45% of the employee's salary, the self-employed individual (who now also happens to be an "employer") withholds $14.50 ($1,000.00 x 1.45%) from the check of the newly hired employee. The employer is then required to match the amount that he or she withheld from the employee. Therefore, the employer must send a total of $29.00 to the IRS for Medicare payments — $14.50 that was withheld from the employee and $14.50 from his or her own pocket.

MEDICARE PART A: BANKRUPT IN 2002

At the same time, the employer will also forward an amount that is required to be withheld as Social Security taxes from the employee. The Social Security withholding rate is 6.20%. So, the employer also withholds $62.00 from the employee's paycheck. The employer must match this amount also.

Finally, the employer is required to withhold income taxes from the employee. This amount can vary, but for the newly hired employee assume that the amount is $150.00. The employer does not match this amount. So every two weeks, the employee gets a check for $773.50, and the employer sends the IRS a check for $303.00 computed as shown below:

	Employee	Employer
Salary	$1,000.00	
Medicare taxes	(14.50)	$29.00
Social Security taxes	(62.00)	124.00
Income taxes	(150.00)	150.00
Net paycheck	$773.50	
Amount sent to IRS		$303.00

By the end of the calendar year, the employee will have paid $348.00 in Medicare Part A taxes, and the employer will have payed $348.00 on behalf of that employee.

The example shown above only satisfies the obligation for the employee's Medicare taxes. The employer is also responsible for Medicare taxes on his or her earnings as a self-employed individual. Unlike the employee, however, the self-employed individual waits until the end of the year to determine his or her earnings for the year.

Assume the self-employed individual had a good year and earned $200,000.00 after paying all of his or her ex-

penses, including the salary and taxes of the employee.
The self-employed individual would file a tax return for
the year showing that he or she owed the following
amounts to the IRS:

Income taxes $50,091.00
  (Married filing jointly, two
  children, no itemized deductions.

Social Security taxes .... $ 7,514.40
  ($60,600.00 x 12.4%)

Medicare taxes .... $ 5,356.30
  ($200,000.00 x 92.35% x 2.9%)

Total taxes owed for 1994 .... $62,961.70

It is important to note two items about the above calculation. First, the self-employed person is responsible
for paying the full 2.9% Medicare rate on his or her earnings. Second, there is a cap on the amount of wages that
are subject to the Social Security tax. For 1994, only the
first $60,600 of earnings were subject to Social Security
taxes. However, as a result of the 1993 tax increase, *there
is no cap on earnings for the Medicare tax.* The self-employed
individual first multiplies his earnings by 92.35% and
then multiplies the product by 2.9% to arrive at the total
Medicare taxes owed. **NO WONDER TALK OF SIMPLIFYING
TAXES IS SO POPULAR THESE DAYS!**
  The removal of the cap on earnings of self-employed
persons as well as employees was an effort by the Clinton
Administration in 1993 to shore up the failing Medicare
Part A trust fund. This tax increase took effect in 1994 as
reflected in the table on page 84. It was some help, but

not enough. Obviously, this was a one-time solution. It now appears that the only way to get more money into the Medicare Part A system under the current structure is to raise the Medicare tax rate above its current 2.9% level.

RISING TAXES

The table on page 84 indicates that the Medicare tax rate and the cap on wages has been steadily rising since 1966 when the Medicare program began.

In the last 30 years, the tax rate has risen from 0.35% to 2.9%. **THE INCREASES WERE NEEDED TO PAY FOR ESCALATING COSTS AND LARGER NUMBERS OF BENEFICIARIES.** Of course, the amount of earned income subject to tax has also increased steadily.

Even though the Medicare Part A tax has risen substantially since the program began in 1966, the program is still a bargain for anyone who is now retired or who will soon retire. The table on page 84 indicates that for a self-employed person who retired at the end of 1993, the maximum amount that he or she would have contributed to the Medicare program was $22,938.70. The amount would have been one-half this amount, or $11,469.35 for an employee who earned the limit during the years of 1966 through 1993. The other half would have been paid by the employer.

INTENSIVE CARE

Medicare Tax Rates and Wages Subject to Tax
for a Self-Employed Individual
1966 through 1995

Year	Maximum taxable amount	Contribution rate	Amount
1966	$6,600	0.35%	$23.10
1967	6,600	0.50%	33.00
1968	7,800	0.60%	46.80
1969	7,800	0.60%	46.80
1970	7,800	0.60%	46.80
1971	7,800	0.60%	46.80
1972	9,000	0.60%	54.00
1973	10,800	1.00%	108.00
1974	13,200	0.90%	118.80
1975	14,100	0.90%	126.90
1976	15,300	0.90%	137.70
1977	16,500	0.90%	148.50
1978	17,700	1.00%	177.00
1979	22,900	1.05%	240.45
1980	25,900	1.05%	271.95
1981	29,700	1.30%	386.10
1982	32,400	1.30%	421.20
1983	35,700	1.30%	464.10
1984	37,800	2.60%	982.80
1985	39,600	2.70%	1,069.20
1986	42,000	2.90%	1,218.00
1987	43,800	2.90%	1,270.20
1988	45,000	2.90%	1,305.00
1989	48,000	2.90%	1,392.00
1990	51,300	2.90%	1,487.70
1991	125,000	2.90%	3,625.00
1992	130,200	2.90%	3,775.80
1993	135,000	2.90%	3,915.00
1994	no limit	2.90%	unlimited
1995	no limit	2.90%	unlimited

TOTAL TAXES PAID (1966-1993)   **$22,938.70**

MEDICARE PART A: BANKRUPT IN 2002

Under the current benefit structure, a person who retired in 1993 will receive more than $2.50 in Medicare
Part A benefits for every dollar he and his employer paid
in Medicare taxes. The average Medicare recipient received about $3,000 in Part A benefits in 1994. At this
rate it will take less than 8 years for a Medicare recipient
to receive benefits worth more than the *maximum* amount
he or she could have been responsible for putting into
the system. A single hospital stay can easily consume this
amount.

RISING TAXES, PART II

The trustees of the Medicare Part A trust fund are also
aware, of course, that the only way to get more money
into the Part A program is to raise the tax rate. According
to their 1995 report, to keep the Hospital Insurance program operating for the next 25 years requires that an additional 1.3% be added to the current 2.9% tax rate. This
would mean an additional 0.65% tax on the employee
and 0.65% tax on the employer. For example, an employee making $100,000 would pay another $650 in taxes
each year.

The Trustees' report goes on to say that the alternative to a tax increase is to cut Medicare spending by 30%
or somehow raise the program's income by 44%. This
would solve the problem until the year 2020, at which
time the tax would have to be raised again. By the year
2050 the tax is expected to triple from its current level.
The chart on page 86 indicates the Trustees' estimates of
the payroll tax rates needed to keep the trust fund sol-
vent from 2005 through 2055.

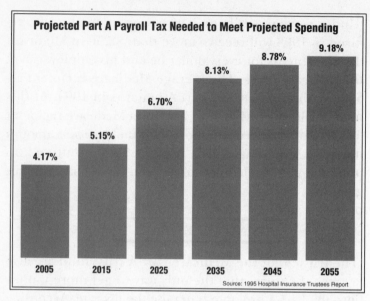

Projected Part A Payroll Tax Needed to Meet Projected Spending

Source: 1995 Hospital Insurance Trustees Report

Americans cannot afford to be taxed more and more to meet the needs of a program that can be modernized to save money. Over the years Medicare spending will have to increase to meet the needs of more eligible beneficiaries and rising health care costs, *but spending will have to increase at an affordable rate.* This does not necessarily mean that taxes will have to be raised. Tax revenue can be increased by putting more people to work in higher paying jobs.

For example, a company with 100 employees each making $20,000 a year will contribute $58,000 to Medicare Part A under the current 2.9% payroll tax. If the payroll tax rate is raised to 3.9%, Medicare would then receive $78,000 in taxes from this company.

Instead of raising taxes, assume that this company will hire 10 new people a year for five years and raise salaries 25% over the five-year period. At the end of this time period there would be 150 employees earning approximately $25,000 each. Under the current 2.9% payroll tax this company and its employees would contribute more than $108,000 to Medicare Part A. The increase of $30,000 is a result of a growing and improving economy, not higher taxes.

This is yet another example of why Medicare reform must be debated as part of the entire budget balancing process. If the budget can be balanced, the economy will grow along with employment and wages. With more people working and making more money, Medicare will receive more money without having to raise taxes.

PAY-AS-YOU-GO

One of the biggest myths associated with Medicare is that the Medicare taxes paid by hard-working men and women are placed in a secure fund to finance their own medical retirement benefits. Medicare is actually a "pay-as-you-go" program. The taxes paid by the workers of today are paying for the benefits received by today's Medicare recipients. The taxes paid years ago by today's retirees have already been spent.

The charts on page 88 show where the income of Medicare Part A came from and where it went in 1994. The combination of these two charts shows that Medicare Part A received $106 billion in 1994 and paid out $103 billion in benefits. As shown on the next page, 86.7% of the financing for Medicare Part A came straight from the payroll tax. As discussed in Chapter 3, this money is not put away somewhere and saved until the workers of today retire.

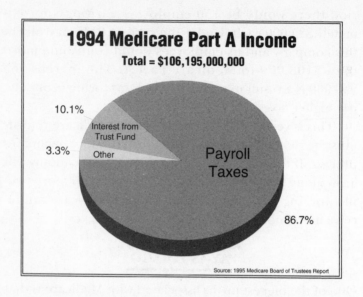

1994 Medicare Part A Income
Total = $106,195,000,000

10.1%
Interest from
Trust Fund

3.3%
Other

Payroll
Taxes

86.7%

Source: 1995 Medicare Board of Trustees Report

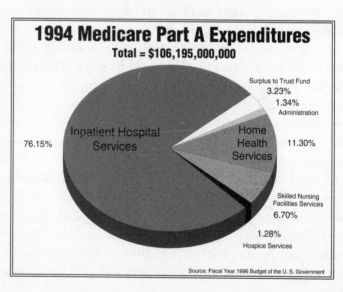

1994 Medicare Part A Expenditures
Total = $106,195,000,000

Surplus to Trust Fund
3.23%

1.34%
Administration

Inpatient Hospital
Services

Home
Health
Services   11.30%

76.15%

Skilled Nursing
Facilities Services
6.70%

1.28%
Hospice Services

Source: Fiscal Year 1996 Budget of the U. S. Government

MEDICARE PART A: BANKRUPT IN 2002

In 1994, the remaining 3.23% surplus was transferred to the Medicare Part A trust fund, which then lent that money to the federal government to be spent on programs that have nothing to do with health care. Instead of raising taxes or cutting spending, the government has spent the money in the trust fund. When Medicare Part A needs the $136 billion that should be in the Medicare Trust Fund in 1996, the *taxpayers* will have to repay the money to the trust fund.

RISING COSTS

As Medicare costs rise, so does the amount of money that Medicare recipients are expected to pay from their own pocket. Medicare Part A does not cover 100% of hospital costs or other expenses. The table on page 90 shows what costs Medicare Part A covers and how much each recipient is expected to pay.

For example, Medicare Part A recipients must pay the first $716 of their hospital bill. Over the years this payment, called a deductible, has been raised from $40 in 1966 to the 1995 level of $716.

Many senior citizens and disabled Medicare beneficiaries cannot afford to pay the expenses that Medicare Part A does not cover. The Medigap insurance policies purchased from private insurance companies that were discussed in Chapter 4, cover a portion and sometimes all of these expenses. However, many beneficiaries cannot afford a Medigap insurance plan.

Today, many hospitals and other health care providers that treat Medicare patients cannot afford to pay hospitals and other health care providers what Medicare does not cover. To make up for this lost revenue, many

INTENSIVE CARE

MEDICARE Part A: 1995			
Services	**Benefit**	**Medicare Pays**	**You Pay**
HOSPITALIZATION			
Semiprivate room and board, general	First 60 days	All but $716	$716
nursing and other hospital services	61st to 90th day	All but $179 a day	$179 a day
and supplies.	91st to 150th day	All but $358 a day	$358 a day
(Medicare payments based on benefit periods.)	Beyond 150 days	Nothing	All costs
SKILLED NURSING FACILITY CARE			
Semiprivate room and board, skilled	First 20 days	100% approved amount.	Nothing
nursing and rehabilitative services	Additional 80 days	All but $89.50 a day	$89.50 a day
and other services and supplies. *(Medicare payments based on benefit periods.)*	Beyond 100 days	Nothing	All costs
HOME HEALTH CARE			
Part-time or intermittent skilled care, home health aid services, durable medical equipment and supplies and other services	Unlimited when Medicare conditions are met.	100% of approved amount; 80% of approved amount for durable medical equipment.	Nothing for services; 20% approved amount for durable medical equipment.

hospitals and other health care providers have been forced to increase their charges on non-Medicare patients who are typically covered by private insurance. This process of cost shifting is legal and in most cases is a matter of financial survival for health care providers.

MEDICARE PATIENTS ACCOUNT FOR APPROXIMATELY ONE-THIRD OF ALL HOSPITAL PATIENTS. HOWEVER, HOSPITALS RECEIVE JUST 24% OF THEIR ANNUAL REVENUE FROM MEDICARE PART A. AS A RESULT, NON-MEDICARE PATIENTS SUBSIDIZE MEDICARE THROUGH COST SHIFTING.

MEDICARE PART A: BANKRUPT IN 2002

If Medicare Part A is not updated to put it on a sound financial footing, every hospital, every patient and every taxpayer will suffer. Rural hospitals, large community hospitals and research hospitals like the Mayo Clinic, all depend on Medicare for a large part of their revenue. Imagine what would happen to the overall quality of health care in America if the financial stability of Medicare cannot be maintained.

This is the direction our health care system is headed. Our elected leaders must act now to stop the out-of-control growth of Medicare.

The bankruptcy of Medicare Part A must be prevented, but saving Part A will not be enough. Rising costs are also threatening Medicare Part B.

6

Medicare Part B: Problems to Solve

The Medicare Part A crisis is serious enough without having any related problems. However, Part A is only 63% of total Medicare spending. Part B, the Supplementary Medical Insurance program that pays for doctor bills and other non-hospital services, comprises the other 37% of Medicare spending.

Medicare Part B is growing at a rate that our country cannot afford. The program is growing even faster than Part A.

MEDICARE PART B HAS GROWN AN AVERAGE OF 15% PER YEAR OVER THE LAST 20 YEARS.

- In the last five years, spending on Medicare Part B has increased a total of 53%.

- Medicare Part B spending grew from $38.3 billion in 1989 to $58.6 billion in 1994.

- **PART B NOW SPENDS 40% MORE ON THE AVERAGE BENEFICIARY THAN IT DID JUST FIVE YEARS AGO.**

INTENSIVE CARE

- **AT ITS CURRENT RATE OF GROWTH, MEDICARE PART B SPENDING WILL DOUBLE IN SIZE EVERY SEVEN YEARS.**

Before discussing the remainder of the Medicare Part B problems, some background information is important.

THE PAYMENT PROCESS

Participation in Medicare Part B is said to be *voluntary*. Anyone over the age of 65 can participate in the program by paying a fee. The fee in 1995 is $46.10 per month. For participants who are receiving Social Security benefits, this fee is automatically deducted from their monthly Social Security check.

In addition to the monthly fee, there are two other types of out-of-pocket costs associated with Medicare Part B. They are called the *deductible* and *coinsurance*. The deductible is the amount of charges for which the patient is responsible each calendar year before his or her Medicare Part B benefits begin. The Medicare Part B deductible is totally separate from the Medicare Part A deductible. In 1995, the Medicare Part B deductible is $100. This means that the patient must pay the first $100 of approved Medicare Part B charges during 1995 before Medicare pays any other bills.

After paying the first $100 of medical costs, the patient is then subject to the coinsurance provision of Medicare Part B. Medicare pays for some, but not all, of the charges for medical services. Medicare will typically pay 80% of a predetermined amount. The patient is responsible for the remainder of the bill.

There are exceptions to the deductible and coinsurance rules for laboratory services, flu shots, and home

MEDICARE PART B: PROBLEMS TO SOLVE

health services. The patient is not usually responsible for any of the cost for these services.

The Medicare program has developed a payment or reimbursement procedure for the health care provider known as the *assignment method*. Under this arrangement, the doctor or supplier agrees to accept the amount approved by Medicare.

Some doctors and suppliers sign agreements to become *Medicare participants*. These doctors and suppliers have agreed to accept the predetermined amount set by the government on all Medicare claims. All health care providers have an opportunity to sign participation agreements each year.

Doctors taking assignment may charge no more than the maximum amount determined by Medicare. Medicare pays the doctor or supplier 80% of the approved amount. The doctor or supplier can charge the Medicare patient only for the remaining 20% of the predetermined amount, assuming the patient's $100 deductible has already been met.

An example will help to explain how the Medicare Part B deductible and coinsurance impact a patient.

- Jim Smith's doctor performed a routine surgical procedure in the office.

- The Medicare-approved charge for the procedure was $400.

- Jim paid $100 of the bill himself to satisfy the deductible for the year.

- Medicare paid $220 [($400 x 80%) - $100 deductible].

- Jim owes another $80.

INTENSIVE CARE

How does Medicare establish the amounts for its approved charges? Without going into great detail, each procedure is ranked according to how much it costs compared to other medical procedures. This *relative value* is then modified to take into account geographical differences because the price of health care varies across the nation. From this formula, Medicare determines the dollar amount for a procedure.

Even if a doctor or supplier is not a Medicare participant, he or she can still treat Medicare patients. For example, many doctors and suppliers may choose to treat only certain Medicare patients. In these situations, Medicare will only pay the doctor 95% of the amount he or she otherwise would have received if he or she had signed a participation agreement.

When a doctor or supplier does not take assignment, he or she is unwilling to accept the Medicare-approved amount as payment in full. So, a bill from a non-participating doctor will usually be higher than a bill from a doctor who agrees to take assignment. For this reason, the patient should always ask a non-participating doctor if he or she will accept the predetermined rate of reimbursement established by Medicare.

If the doctor or supplier does not accept the predetermined rate of reimbursement established by Medicare, the Medicare patient must pay the doctor or supplier directly. After the patient pays the doctor or supplier, Medicare only reimburses the patient for 80% of the predetermined amount, after subtracting any part of the $100 annual deductible that has not been met by the patient.

Doctors, suppliers, and other providers of Part B services must, in most cases, submit Medicare claims for the

MEDICARE PART B: PROBLEMS TO SOLVE

patient. After the Part B claim is processed, Medicare will send the patient a notice labeled *Explanation of Your Medicare Part B Benefits* that will explain how much of the bill is covered by Medicare Part B.

This brief description of the Medicare payment process does not begin to address the problems encountered by doctors and other providers in dealing with the Medicare claims processing system. The time and paperwork involved is enormous. It is probably fair to say that any office consisting of at least two doctors in private practice requires the equivalent of at least one full-time employee to handle Medicare claim forms. Medicare does not pay for this employee. The patients with health care insurance ultimately pay for this paperwork through cost shifting.

COVERED SERVICES

Medicare Part B offers coverage that complements the coverage provided by Part A. The items covered by Medicare Part B are doctors' services, other medical and health services, and home health services. Generally speaking, Medicare Part B covers these costs:

DOCTORS' SERVICES

- Surgery

- Consultation

- Home, office, and institutional visits

- Certain limitations apply for services by dentists, podiatrists, and chiropractors

INTENSIVE CARE

- Certain limitations apply for the treatment of mental illness

OTHER MEDICAL AND HEALTH SERVICES

- Laboratory and other diagnostic tests
- X-ray and radiation therapy
- Outpatient services at a hospital
- Rural health clinic services
- Home dialysis supplies and equipment
- Artificial devices (other than dental)
- Physical and speech therapy
- Ambulance services
- Durable medical equipment

HOME HEALTH SERVICES

- An unlimited number of necessary home health visits for patients not covered under Medicare Part A
- No deductible or coinsurance payments required, except for durable medical equipment

Medicare Part B will also cover second opinions. In fact, it is recommended that the patient get a second opinion before undergoing any type of surgery. If the first and second opinions differ, Medicare Part B will pay for a third opinion as well.

MEDICARE PART B: PROBLEMS TO SOLVE

The table on page 100 shows the categories covered by Medicare Part B and how much each recipient is expected to pay.

Medicare Part B does not pay for:

- Most routine physical examinations
- Routine foot and dental care
- Hearing aids
- Eyeglasses
- Most immunizations
- Most prescription drugs

As mentioned earlier the Medicare Part B costs are growing at an extraordinary rate. The chart below shows

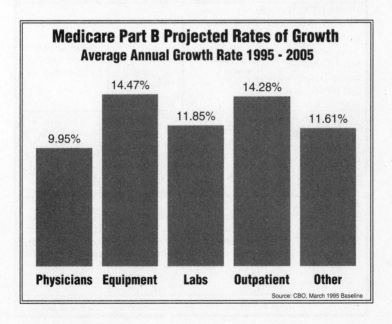

Medicare Part B Projected Rates of Growth
Average Annual Growth Rate 1995 - 2005

Physicians	Equipment	Labs	Outpatient	Other
9.95%	14.47%	11.85%	14.28%	11.61%

Source: CBO, March 1995 Baseline

INTENSIVE CARE

MEDICARE Part B: 1995			
Services	**Benefit**	**Medicare Pays**	**You Pay**
MEDICAL EXPENSES			
Doctor's services, inpatient and outpatient medical and surgical services and supplies, physical and speech therapy, diagnostic tests, durable medical equipment and other services.	Unlimited if medically necessary.	80% approved amount (*after $100 deductible*). Reduced to 50% for most outpatient mental health services.	100% deductible, plus 20% of approved amount and limited charges above approved amount.
CLINICAL LABORATORY SERVICES			
Blood tests, urinalyses, and more.	Unlimited if medically necessary.	Generally 100% of approved amount.	Nothing for services.
HOME HEALTH CARE			
Part-time or intermittent skilled care, home health aide services, durable medical equipment and supplies and other services.	Unlimited as long as you meet Medicare conditions.	100% approved amount; 80% approved amount durable medical equipment.	Nothing for services; 20% of approved amount durable medical equipment.
OUTPATIENT HOSPITAL TREATMENT			
Services for the diagnosis or treatment of illness or injury.	Unlimited if medically necessary.	Medicare payment to hospital based on hospital costs.	20% of billed amount (after $100 deductible).
BLOOD			
	Unlimited if medically necessary.	80% approved amount (after $100 deductible and on 4th pint).	First 3 pints plus 20% of approved amount for additional pints (after $100 deductible).
1995 Part B monthly premium: $46.10 (*Premium may be higher if you enroll late*).			

the average annual growth rate of each particular cost category for the years 1995 through 2005. Each cost category is growing at a rate well beyond inflation.

A CALL TO ACTION

Secretary of the Treasury Robert Rubin, Secretary of Labor Robert Reich, Secretary of Health and Human Services Donna Shalala, and the other Medicare Trustees recognize the danger of this accelerated growth in Medicare Part B spending. They published this warning in the 1995 Trustees' Report for Medicare Part B:

> *The Trustees note with great concern the past and projected rapid growth in the cost of the program.... Growth rates have been so rapid that outlays of the program have increased 53% in aggregate and 40% per enrollee in the last five years.... The Trustees believe that prompt, effective and decisive action is necessary.*

The Trustees' call to action should be taken seriously. Our government should take the necessary steps to halt the skyrocketing spending of Medicare Part B. The citizens of this country should encourage their elected leaders to support viable measures to control this spending. Otherwise, a major warning signal will have been ignored, and this program will continue on its dangerous course.

A "SOUND" PROGRAM?

Despite their warnings about the problems with Medicare Part B, the Trustees were able to conclude that the program was financially "sound." However, the same Trustees referred to Medicare Part A as "out of financial balance." This makes no sense when the costs of both programs are going through the roof. The reason for the difference is that the two programs use different accounting procedures. *The same rules should apply to both programs.*

The accounting procedure that rates the Medicare Part B program as "sound" is based upon *total* income tax receipts by the government. Using this standard, as long as the money flowing into the federal government from income taxes appears to exceed the costs of the Medicare Part B program, the Trustees can declare the program to be "sound."

Under this definition, any government program with an annual cost of approximately $600 billion — the total income tax receipts of the United States for 1995 — would be "sound." Does this make any sense?

Obviously, this is not a good test because income tax receipts are also used to fund other programs and interest on the national debt. The more tax revenues being spent by Medicare Part B, the less money there is for other government programs. Medicare Part B is already demanding a larger percentage of taxpayer revenue than its founders ever intended, and its costs are escalating every year. This definition of "sound" should have been added to the deceptive terms described in Chapter 3.

SAME FORECAST: CLEARLY NOT SUSTAINABLE

Even though the Trustees used different accounting techniques to measure the fiscal health of Part A and Part B, they came to the same conclusion for each program — the programs clearly are not sustainable in their current forms. Our elected leaders should listen to the trustees:

MEDICARE PART B: PROBLEMS TO SOLVE

Given the past and projected cost of the program, the
Trustees urge the Congress to take additional actions
designed to more effectively control SMI (Medicare
Part B) costs through specific program legislation . . .

The Trustees have called for action for many years
now, yet our government does not answer the call. We
must have the foresight to implement change now. Every
day that goes by only makes the problem worse.

BAD PLANNING

The 1966 Medicare Part B program was very different
than the current program. In 1966, Medicare Part B participants paid for approximately 50% of the program
costs through their monthly premiums. The taxpayers
paid the remaining costs. That was how the financing of
Medicare Part B was expected to work.

- As the first chart on page 104 indicates, the
  amount paid by beneficiaries in 1995 covers only
  28% of the cost of Medicare Part B.

- By the year 2004, beneficiaries will pay only 17%
  of the total cost of Medicare Part B.

- **THE REMAINING 83% OF THE COST WILL COME
  FROM THE TAXPAYERS.**

The authors of the original Medicare legislation did
not foresee the changes in population and technology
that would occur in our country. Today, new medical
treatments and increased use of medical services have
created a surge in medical costs and Medicare spending.

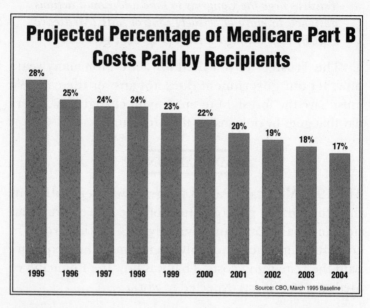

Projected Percentage of Medicare Part B Costs Paid by Recipients

28% 25% 24% 24% 23% 22% 20% 19% 18% 17%

1995 1996 1997 1998 1999 2000 2001 2002 2003 2004

Source: CBO, March 1995 Baseline

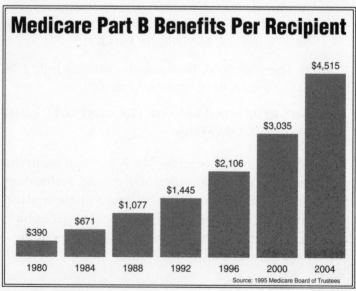

Medicare Part B Benefits Per Recipient

$4,515

$3,035

$2,106

$1,445

$1,077

$671

$390

1980 1984 1988 1992 1996 2000 2004

Source: 1995 Medicare Board of Trustees

MEDICARE PART B: PROBLEMS TO SOLVE

As the bottom chart on page 104 indicates, the average amount received each year by a Medicare Part B recipient has grown dramatically. This spending pattern will only continue until steps are taken to modernize the program. The taxpayers cannot afford this substantial unfunded increase in benefits every year.

We cannot continue to depend on short-term solutions to solve the Medicare Part B spending problems. Band-Aids will not make the Medicare problem go away. The only way to cure this problem is to perform major surgery.

We must implement a long-term plan to contain the overall growth of Medicare spending. Chapter 7 proposes some answers for controlling this runaway growth.

If we do not act soon, Medicare will move from intensive care to critical care.

FOR EXAMPLE, BY THE YEAR 2030, INCREASES IN PART B SPENDING ALONE WILL REQUIRE INCOME TAX INCREASES OF 40%.

WE CANNOT PLACE THIS BURDEN ON OUR CHILDREN AND GRANDCHILDREN.

7

Medicare: Solving the Problems

The basic structure of the Medicare program has remained fundamentally unchanged for 30 years. However, in those same 30 years, our country has experienced sweeping technological, demographic, political, and financial transformations. No business could survive for three decades without adapting to significant changes in the marketplace. Although Medicare is a government program and not a profit-driven business, it exists within the largest single sector of our economy — the health care industry. The enormous size of the Medicare program affects the quality and the cost of health care for everyone.

Countless changes have occurred in private health care plans over the past 30 years. Most of these changes resulted from rapidly rising health care costs. New and innovative systems for delivering health care services have succeeded in slowing the rate of increase in health care costs for the private sector. These changes are, in part, the result of financial incentives offered to participants in various employer health care plans.

Rather than relying on market forces, Medicare attempts to control its costs by imposing limitations on the amounts that doctors and suppliers may charge. In a sector of the economy as large as the health care industry, an artificial limitation of market forces contributes to inefficiency, waste, fraud, and abuse.

Reform is needed, and informed officials in Washington agree.

> *If we don't fix Medicare, there will be no care.*
>
> Rep. John Kasich
> Chairman, House Budget
> Committee

> *One thing is for certain, postponing decisions about Medicare's financing will only make the necessary policy actions in the future more severe.*
>
> June O'Neill
> Director of the Congres-
> sional Budget Office

> *It is not a new issue, but candidly it's time for action.*
>
> David Walker
> Public Trustee
> Social Security and Medi-
> care Boards of Trustees

No one seriously disputes the dimensions of the financial crisis facing the Medicare program. There is broad, bipartisan recognition of the extent of the problem. Some combination of changes and additions to the existing program are needed. For this reason, it is very important for the American public to understand the various Medicare reform proposals that are under discussion.

The health care system in the United States is far too complicated for anyone or any group to claim that a single reform proposal is *the* solution to the crisis. Rather than taking a huge first step with a new untested system, wouldn't it make sense to pilot test a number of proposals? This is the only reasonable method to determine what works and what doesn't work. The danger with scrapping an old system of any kind is that a new system may not be any better.

Past attempts at reforming the Medicare program have seldom succeeded in lowering expenses for very long. Historical data indicate that after reform measures are introduced, costs decline for a brief time. However, within a short while, they begin to increase once again. So, while it is possible to lower the momentary level of spending from time to time, decreasing the rate of growth over a long period of time is a stubborn problem. Any reform proposal must be measured by its ability to produce a lasting decline in the rate of growth currently experienced in the Medicare program.

This chapter describes two approaches to reform: a short-term approach and a long-term approach. The short-term option is designed as a bridge to get from the current system to a new system. The long-term option is designed to introduce a new system and bring about fundamental change in the Medicare program. As mentioned above, fundamental change needs to be approached with caution. This two-step technique would preserve the structure of the current Medicare program while gradually introducing a new plan.

INTENSIVE CARE

The next section of this chapter will discuss some short-term reform proposals designed to correct certain deficiencies of the current Medicare system. These proposals will also recommend methods to reduce waste, fraud, and abuse in the current system.

The last section of the chapter will introduce programs for long-term reform. These programs are relevant not only to Medicare, but Medicaid and the entire health care industry as well. For that reason, these long-term reform proposals will be discussed only briefly in this chapter. Chapter 10 and Chapter 11 address these reform proposals in more detail.

REFORMS TO CURRENT SYSTEM

Today's Medicare system is primarily a "fee-for-service" arrangement. There is little incentive for the beneficiary or the health care provider to be cost conscious. As a result of the 20% coinsurance provision of Part B, Medicare recipients are only paying 20 cents of every health care dollar they use. The taxpayers are paying the other 80 cents. This is at least part of the reason that Medicare spending has soared.

This chapter presents a number of short-term reform proposals. Some of these ideas can be traced to a particular source. In these cases, the originator of the idea is noted. Other proposals have evolved over time, and it is difficult to determine the original developer. In these cases, the most recent source of the information is noted.

MEDICARE: SOLVING THE PROBLEMS

RAISING COST AWARENESS

To address the problems presented by the "fee-for-service" structure, members of Congress do not have to look very far. The Congressional Budget Office (CBO) has suggested a series of possible reforms that would provide an incentive to Medicare participants to control spending.

INCREASING THE DEDUCTIBLE

As discussed in Chapter 6, the Medicare Part B deductible is the amount the patient must pay for services each year before the government begins to cover 80% of the patient's bills. The deductible was set at $50 in 1966, and has been increased only three times since then. As unbelievable as it seems, Medicare patients in 1967 averaged $111 *per year* in doctor bills. The average patient was paying almost one half of his or her annual medical costs as a result of the deductible.

SINCE 1970 THE AMOUNT SPENT BY THE FEDERAL GOVERNMENT FOR HEALTH CARE INCREASED ALMOST 2,100%. BUT THE AMOUNT OF THE DEDUCTIBLE HAS ONLY INCREASED 100% — FROM $50 TO $100.

In 1995, the deductible accounts for only 5% of the average patient's Medicare Part B costs for the year.

In 1966, the deductible had the effect of forcing a patient to consider whether a trip to the doctor was really necessary — at least until the deductible had been met for the year. In 1995 the deductible is more of a nuisance than anything else. The patient usually meets the deductible in the first one or two doctor visits each year. After that, the patient is spending 20 cents and the government is spending 80 cents for every health care dollar that beneficiaries spend.

INTENSIVE CARE

The CBO suggests increasing the deductible to $150 in 1996, and then indexing it to the rate of growth in the Medicare program. Raising the deductible would increase cost consciousness because the patient would pay for more services out of his or her own pocket. It would also lower the taxpayers' share of the cost of Medicare. **THE CBO ESTIMATES THAT THIS REFORM PROPOSAL WOULD SAVE $15.2 BILLION OVER SEVEN YEARS.**

EXPANDING COINSURANCE

Under the current Medicare system, coinsurance payments are not required for laboratory services, home health services and skilled nursing facilities. Medicare pays for 100% of these services. In Medicare Part B, there is a 20% co-payment on almost all other services. Adding the requirement of a 20% co-payment to these three services would save money for the taxpayers in two ways. First, it would reduce the amount the government pays for these services. Second, it might reduce the utilization of the service when the Medicare recipient realizes there is a cost associated with them. **THE CBO ESTIMATES THE TOTAL PROJECTED SAVINGS FROM THIS PLAN WOULD BE $28.3 BILLION OVER FIVE YEARS.**

REFORMING MEDIGAP

Medigap policies are the insurance policies that provide coverage for the items not paid by the Medicare program. Analysts believe that Medigap policies have the effect of encouraging overuse of services. As long as the Medicare recipient has already paid the premium for the Medigap policy, there is no additional cost to the recipient to using the services covered under the policy.

MEDICARE: SOLVING THE PROBLEMS

In order to control Medicare costs, the Medigap problem must be addressed in reform proposals. This coverage pays for all or most of the Medicare co-payment requirements. **STUDIES INDICATE THAT MEDIGAP POLICYHOLDERS USE ABOUT 24% MORE SERVICES THAN THEY WOULD IF THEY DID NOT HAVE THIS SO-CALLED *FIRST-DOLLAR COVERAGE*.** When Medicare beneficiaries use additional services, the taxpayers end up paying for most of the costs.

The above description is not intended to be an indictment of Medicare beneficiaries or an exposé of their spending habits. It merely points out the results of studies seeking answers to questions about the rising costs of Medicare.

One solution to the overuse of services might be to prohibit Medigap plans from offering first-dollar coverage for Medicare's co-payment requirements. For example, in 1996, Medigap plans could be prohibited from paying any portion of the first $1,500 of a policy holder's annual co-payment requirements. In later years, the Medigap limit could be linked to growth in the average value of Medicare's co-payment requirements. **THE CBO ESTIMATES THAT SAVINGS FROM THIS PROPOSAL WOULD TOTAL $34.9 BILLION OVER FIVE YEARS.**

REDUCING THE SUBSIDY

The Congressional Budget Office has also proposed several reform measures that are designed to reduce the amount the taxpayers must pay to subsidize the cost of the Medicare Part B program.

INTENSIVE CARE

RAISING PREMIUMS

There are many reform proposals regarding the Medicare Part B premium. Chapter 6 explained that the Part B premium, paid by beneficiaries, was initially intended to cover 50% of the cost of benefits. However, the premiums paid by Medicare recipients now only pay for 28% of Part B services. The other 72% of the costs are covered by the taxpayers and increased deficit spending.

The 1993 budget act requires that the Medicare Part B premium be set at 25% of costs in 1996. This leaves taxpayers paying for 75% of the cost of the program. For this reason, various reform proposals attempt to decrease the percentage of government funding for Medicare Part B.

One proposal would increase the Part B premium for new beneficiaries who choose the typical fee-for-service alternative instead of a new, more cost effective health care plan. Beginning in 1999, all *new* beneficiaries choosing Medicare fee-for-service would pay $20 more in Part B premiums than current Medicare participants. Current beneficiaries would not have to pay the higher premium. **THE CBO ESTIMATES SAVINGS FROM THIS PROPOSAL WOULD BE $3.8 BILLION OVER SEVEN YEARS.**

Another proposal would increase the Part B premium to cover 30% of the program cost in 1996 and every year thereafter. The premium for 1996 would be $54 a month instead of the current $46.10 per month. **THE CBO ESTIMATES THAT THIS PROPOSAL WOULD SAVE $26.3 BILLION OVER FIVE YEARS.**

One more option in connection with the Part B premium is a return to the initial 50/50 split between the Medicare recipient and the government. This plan, proposed by the Heritage Foundation, would limit the federal government to 50% of the Part B spending. If this change had been in effect in 1995, the premium would have been $92.20 per month. This increase would be a hardship for many lower income participants. **IT IS ESTIMATED THAT THIS PREMIUM INCREASE WOULD SAVE AS MUCH AS $121.5 BILLION OVER FIVE YEARS.**

INCREASING AGE OF ELIGIBILITY

This reform proposal is usually discussed in relation to increasing the age of eligibility for Social Security benefits. However, because of the close relationship between Social Security and Medicare, the same type of reform proposal is being suggested for Medicare. In the mid-1930s, when the retirement age for Social Security was established at age 65, the average life expectancy was about 60 years. Today, it is 76.

There are many different ways the Medicare eligibility age could be changed in response to this increased life expectancy. One proposal is for the eligibility age to gradually rise from 65 to 68. This process would begin in 1996, increasing by three months each year until it reached age 68 in the year 2007. The eligibility age will have risen by only three years, compared with a life expectancy increase of 16 years since the eligibility age was first established in the 1930s. This three-year increase would significantly lower the number of Medicare beneficiaries and create substantial savings.

MEANS TESTING PART B

An often discussed reform proposal is to apply a so-called *means test* to Medicare Part B premiums for upper-income beneficiaries. Under this proposal, a Medicare beneficiary would pay a higher premium as his or her income rises.

INTENSIVE CARE

Several different levels of income have been proposed for Part B means testing. One version is that individuals with income of less than $50,000 and couples with income lower than $65,000 would pay a premium that is based upon 25% of the program costs. Premiums would rise progressively for higher-income participants. The maximum premium would cover 50% of costs for individuals with income exceeding $60,000 and for couples with income exceeding $80,000. **THE CBO ESTIMATES THIS OPTION WOULD SAVE $13.9 BILLION OVER FIVE YEARS.**

ELIMINATING WASTE AND OVERPAYMENT

An extensive amount of waste, fraud, and abuse occurs within the Medicare program. The following reform proposals are designed to deal with some of the trouble spots.

MERGING PART A AND PART B

For reforms to have a lasting impact on the Medicare program, the system must be completely reexamined in relation to the current health care environment. When the Medicare program was enacted in 1965, it was divided into Part A and Part B. At that time, the vast majority of important health care procedures occurred in hospitals so this portion of Medicare was placed into a separate program.

Since 1965, the role of the hospital has changed. Many more services are now provided in doctors' offices, surgical centers, clinical labs, and diagnostic centers. Now that hospitals share many of their services with these other providers, the reason for dividing Medicare into two parts should be reconsidered.

Having two independent parts of Medicare has complicated past attempts at reform. Many changes have simply shifted costs from Part A to Part B, and vice versa. If the two parts of Medicare were integrated, it would be easier to assess the impact of reforms on the overall Medicare program.

The combination of Part A and Part B would make the administration of the program much more efficient. Having one bureaucracy instead of two would also save money.

Beyond the administrative efficiencies, combining Part A and Part B would resolve the confusion about the future of Medicare. As discussed in the preceding chapters, funding for Part A and Part B comes from different sources. Presumably there was some logic in 1965 behind handling the financing of Part A and Part B in such a diverse manner. It hardly seems sensible to continue the practice today. This is particularly true given that Part A has been described by the Medicare Trustees as "out of financial balance," while Part B has been described by the same individuals as "sound."

REWARDING HONESTY

Faulty billings that result in overpayments to health care providers is a problem in the Medicare program. This problem is partially due to the lack of an incentive on the part of the Medicare patient to monitor the cost of services he or she receives. To create an incentive, this reform proposal would pay 10% of the savings to a Medicare recipient who detected and reported an overcharging situation. This would result in a more cost-effective system, a more careful billing process, and a reward for alert Medicare beneficiaries.

INTENSIVE CARE

ELIMINATING BAD DEBT PAYMENTS

As previously noted, Medicare beneficiaries are responsible for certain deductible and coinsurance payments when they receive hospital services. If the patient fails to make these payments, the hospital will take action to collect the bill. Under current regulations, if the hospital makes a reasonable effort to collect these amounts and still does not receive payment, Medicare will fully reimburse the hospital for any unpaid amounts. Because Medicare will eventually pay anyway, hospitals sometimes do not conduct as thorough a collection effort as might otherwise be warranted. As a result, bad debt claims have more than doubled since the inception of this policy.

This proposal would eliminate the payments for the bad debts of Medicare recipients. Without Medicare's reimbursement, hospitals would have a financial incentive to expand their collection attempts. **THE CBO ESTIMATES THE SAVINGS FROM THIS REFORM PROPOSAL TO BE $2.7 BILLION OVER SEVEN YEARS.**

REDUCING OR ELIMINATING DISPROPORTIONATE SHARE PAYMENTS

The Medicare program provides for higher reimbursement rates to be paid to hospitals with a disproportionately large share of low-income patients. This extra compensation is called a *disproportionate share payment*. In 1985, Congress added this adjustment to account for the low income Medicare patients who may be more expensive to treat. However, hospital cost data provide only limited support that these payments are justified. More than 1,900 hospitals receive disproportionate share payments, but only 160 large urban hospitals actually have high rates of treating needy patients.

MEDICARE: SOLVING THE PROBLEMS

If the disproportionate share payments were eliminated immediately, the CBO estimates $22.4 billion could be saved over five years. Phasing out the disproportionate share payments by the end of the year 2000 would save approximately $13.4 billion over five years. Another option would be to cut disproportionate share payments for all hospitals except the large urban institutions that treat the most low income patients. **IF THE PAYMENTS WERE ONLY GIVEN TO THOSE HOSPITALS AND LOWERED TO 5%, SAVINGS FOR THE FIVE-YEAR PERIOD WOULD BE ABOUT $21.9 BILLION ACCORDING TO THE CBO.**

REDUCING DIRECT EDUCATION COSTS

Medicare currently makes separate payments to hospitals for the direct costs of providing graduate medical education. These reimbursements pay for the salaries and benefits of the residents, the teaching costs, and the institutional overhead. This reform proposal would reduce teaching and overhead payments for residents, but it would continue to pay the salaries and fringe benefits of the residents. **THE CBO ESTIMATES THIS CHANGE WOULD SAVE $6.1 BILLION OVER SEVEN YEARS.**

This reform proposal is a good example of a situation where cost shifting might occur. For example, if a county hospital lost Medicare money as a result of this reform, local property taxes might have to be increased to make up the difference.

Another potential problem will be the effect this cutback has on the quality of teaching. Reforms like this must be closely scrutinized and pilot tested to avoid injuring the medical system.

INTENSIVE CARE

REDUCING INDIRECT EDUCATION COSTS

Indirect teaching costs consist of factors contributing to higher expenses in medical teaching programs. Reasons for these higher costs include a large population of severely ill patients, an inner city location, more frequent tests and procedures, and more costly staff and facilities. All of these factors are associated with large teaching programs, and they add extra costs. In order to compensate for these indirect teaching costs, payments to the teaching hospitals are increased according to the number of interns and residents on staff.

The General Accounting Office and Prospective Payment Assessment Commission of Medicare have both found that the annual compensation to these hospitals for indirect teaching costs is too high. This proposal would lower the extra Medicare payments to these hospitals. **THE CHANGE WOULD GENERATE $21.1 BILLION IN SAVINGS OVER SEVEN YEARS ACCORDING TO THE CBO.**

LIMITING PAYMENTS TO COSTLY HOSPITAL DOCTORS

Some doctors in hospitals charge much higher amounts per patient than doctors in other hospitals. In order to help modify this disparity, this proposal would reduce payments to hospitals that pay doctors unusually high amounts. The purpose would be to encourage the doctors in these hospitals to reduce their fees. If they do reduce their fees in the year the fees are withheld, Medicare will pay the doctor some or all of the amount of money withheld. **THE CBO ESTIMATES THIS REFORM WOULD SAVE $6 BILLION OVER SEVEN YEARS.**

BEYOND MEDICARE REFORM
TO LONG-TERM REFORM

The preceding discussion of reform possibilities *is not* intended to be a comprehensive inventory of every Medicare reform proposal. It is more of a catalogue of some of the ideas that are beginning to appear with increasing frequency.

As mentioned at the beginning of this chapter, fixing the Medicare program as it exists today is a short-term solution, but it cannot be a long-term answer. As long as neither the patient nor the health care provider has much of an incentive to control costs, the above reform proposals are just like putting more patches on a leaky inner tube.

It will take a fundamental long-term change of some type to truly make a difference. The most promising approach to lasting reform is to introduce the element of choice for Medicare beneficiaries. The best alternative for reform is *not* a "one-size-fits-all" plan. Rather, the key to the future of Medicare is to offer a program that allows a recipient to choose from a variety of plans.

Giving Medicare recipients the freedom to choose from a menu of plans will bring a level of competition to the health care market that is missing at this time. Many of these plans generally fall under the category of so-called *managed care* options. These plans will be discussed in Chapter 10.

Broadening the options for the delivery of health care services to Medicare recipients is a big step on the road to long-term reform. However, complete reform of the Medicare program will also require reform of the Medicare financing system. One of the most interesting financing innovations in the overall health care industry is the

Medical Savings Account (MSA). If, in fact, the health care industry is capable of functioning in a free-market environment, then MSAs could be the key to a true system of choice. MSAs will be discussed in Chapter 11.

The concept of choice as an approach to long-term reform of the Medicare program can probably best be explained with the diagram below.

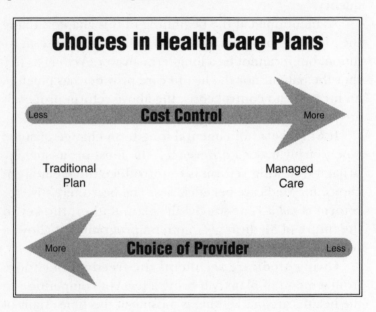

Choices in Health Care Plans

Less   **Cost Control**   More

Traditional Plan   Managed Care

More   **Choice of Provider**   Less

The diagram indicates that controlling costs means less freedom in the choice of health care providers. But less freedom does not imply a lower quality of health care.

ANY REFORM PROPOSAL SHOULD ALLOW MEDICARE BENEFICIARIES TO CHOOSE THE TYPE OF HEALTH CARE PLAN THEY PREFER. THE CHOICE AMONG A TRADITIONAL FEE-FOR-SERVICE PLAN, A MANAGED CARE PLAN, OR ANY PLAN IN BETWEEN SHOULD BE MADE BY THE PATIENT, NOT THE GOVERNMENT.

8

Medicaid: The Last Safety Net

Reforming Medicare is only part of the federal health care battle. Its sound-alike twin, Medicaid, is also in need of an overhaul. Like Medicare, Medicaid was enacted in 1965 to offer health care to millions of Americans who did not have the means to pay for their own care. While Medicare was created to help senior citizens, Medicaid was established to help the needy.

There is no doubt Medicaid has benefited our society. The millions of families who struggle to even put food on their table now have a sense of security knowing they can receive quality health care. This is something the United States should be proud of and continue to support. A great nation like ours has a responsibility to assist those who need help.

As the previous chapters have explained, health care is not inexpensive. **TO CARE FOR THE 33 MILLION PEOPLE WHO MEDICAID WILL COVER IN 1995, THE PROGRAM WILL**

SPEND APPROXIMATELY $156 BILLION. Unlike Medicare, this enormous bill is shared by the federal government *and* each of the state governments. Even the District of Columbia and American territories like Guam and Puerto Rico pay a share.

The chart below shows expected state, federal and total spending on Medicaid from 1995 to 2005. As Medicaid continues to grow out of control, it will consume more federal, state and even local funds.

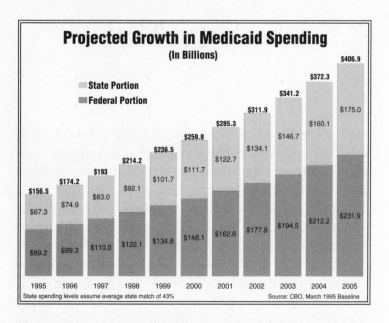

Projected Growth in Medicaid Spending
(In Billions)

■ State Portion
■ Federal Portion

Year	Total	State Portion	Federal Portion
1995	$156.5	$67.3	$89.2
1996	$174.2	$74.9	$99.3
1997	$193	$83.0	$110.0
1998	$214.2	$92.1	$122.1
1999	$236.5	$101.7	$134.8
2000	$259.8	$111.7	$148.1
2001	$285.3	$122.7	$162.6
2002	$311.9	$134.1	$177.8
2003	$341.2	$146.7	$194.5
2004	$372.3	$160.1	$212.2
2005	$406.9	$175.0	$231.9

State spending levels assume average state match of 43%   Source: CBO, March 1995 Baseline

This program is having a much more widespread effect than Medicare on states and municipalities. If costs are not controlled, governments in towns like Peoria to state capitals like Sacramento to Washington, D.C. will be forced to cut other important programs to pay for Medicaid.

MEDICAID: THE LAST SAFETY NET

MANY PROGRAMS, SAME PROBLEMS

One of the most unique aspects of the Medicaid system is that it is actually 56 separate programs. States, territories and the District of Columbia are in charge of administering their own Medicaid programs. The federal government just serves as a manager, overseeing the state programs and setting certain guidelines.

The federal government ends up paying a large part of the Medicaid bill.

IN 1995 THE FEDERAL GOVERNMENT WILL PAY AP-PROXIMATELY 57%, OR $89 BILLION, OF THE TOTAL SPENDING ON MEDICAID.

As the chart below shows, no other major federal expenditure is growing faster.

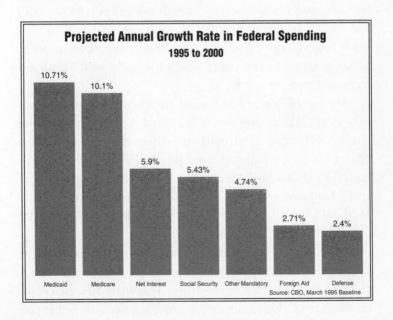

Projected Annual Growth Rate in Federal Spending
1995 to 2000

Medicaid	10.71%
Medicare	10.1%
Net Interest	5.9%
Social Security	5.43%
Other Mandatory	4.74%
Foreign Aid	2.71%
Defense	2.4%

Source: CBO, March 1995 Baseline

INTENSIVE CARE

- **FOR THE NEXT 10 YEARS THE FEDERAL COST OF MEDICAID IS EXPECTED TO RISE ABOUT 11% EACH YEAR.**

- **FEDERAL SPENDING ON MEDICAID WILL INCREASE FROM $89 BILLION IN 1995 TO OVER $231 BILLION IN THE YEAR 2005 — AN INCREASE OF OVER 250%.**

The federal government is not alone in dealing with increasing Medicaid payments. Spending by the states is also escalating too fast.

- **MEDICAID SPENDING BY THE STATES WILL ALSO INCREASE BY MORE THAN 250% — FROM $67 BILLION IN 1995 TO $175 BILLION IN 2005.**

Rising Medicaid payments usually have a greater effect on state budgets than the federal budget. Most states are forced by law to live within their means because they must balance their budgets. As a result, spending in other areas must be cut to make room for increased Medicaid expenditures.

Medicaid is already one of the most expensive state programs. According to the National Association of State Budget Officers, Medicaid spending is expected to account for 20% of all state budgets in 1995. The graph on page 127 shows how Medicaid has increased its portion of state budgets over the years. In comparison, federal Medicaid spending is expected to be about 5.8% of total federal spending in 1995.

The federal government reacts to increasing budget pressures differently than the states. When spending increases, the federal government usually just borrows more money. This is an irresponsible practice, but it can

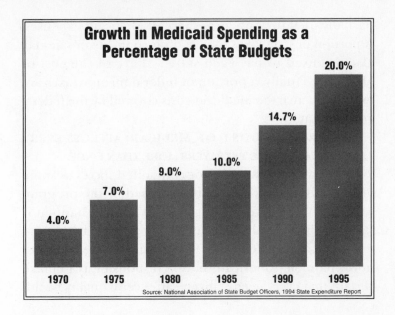

Growth in Medicaid Spending as a Percentage of State Budgets

- 1970: 4.0%
- 1975: 7.0%
- 1980: 9.0%
- 1985: 10.0%
- 1990: 14.7%
- 1995: 20.0%

Source: National Association of State Budget Officers, 1994 State Expenditure Report

ultimately benefit the states. As discussed later in this chapter, many states have become experts at raising federal Medicaid funds and spending the money for other purposes. Medicaid constitutes 40% of all aid that states receive from Washington. With this much money at stake, some states have found ways to manipulate the system.

In some states money for Medicaid is collected at the local level. Many states require local governments and hospitals to pay a portion of Medicaid expenses. Whether by specific taxes on hospitals or by a direct contribution, municipalities are also suffering from the burden of rising Medicaid costs.

With Medicaid funding coming from so many different sources, it is possible for a taxpayer to contribute to the cost of Medicaid through taxes at all three levels of government. Local taxes such as property taxes can be partially used to pay a local share of Medicaid expenses. A portion of state taxes such as an income tax or sales tax also are used to pay each state's share of the cost of Medicaid. Finally, a portion of federal income taxes are used to finance the Medicaid costs covered by the federal government.

THE RISING COST OF MEDICAID AFFECTS EVERY TAXPAYER AND SOME TAXPAYERS MORE THAN ONCE.

If Medicaid costs are not controlled, taxes at some level or all levels will have to be raised or the program will have to be severely cut back. What will happen if states or the federal government – or possibly both – can no longer afford Medicaid? This is a nightmare that must never happen. Americans have a responsibility to make certain that every needy citizen can receive quality health care.

WHO GETS MEDICAID?

For millions of Americans who live in poverty, Medicaid is their sole source of health care. Combined federal and state spending makes Medicaid the largest payer of health care for the needy. The chart on page 129 shows the health care coverage for the needy. Over 48% of Americans who live in poverty depend on Medicaid to pay for their health care needs.

- **IN 1995, 33 MILLION PEOPLE WILL RELY ON MEDICAID FOR EVERYTHING FROM CHILDBIRTH TO NURSING HOME CARE.**

- **MEDICAID HELPS FINANCE HEALTH CARE FOR MORE THAN ONE OUT OF EVERY TEN AMERICANS.**

MEDICAID: THE LAST SAFETY NET

- ONE OUT OF EVERY FOUR AMERICAN CHILDREN DEPENDS ON MEDICAID FOR HIS OR HER BASIC CARE, SUCH AS IMMUNIZATION SHOTS.

- ONE-THIRD OF ALL BIRTHS IN THE UNITED STATES ARE PAID FOR BY MEDICAID.

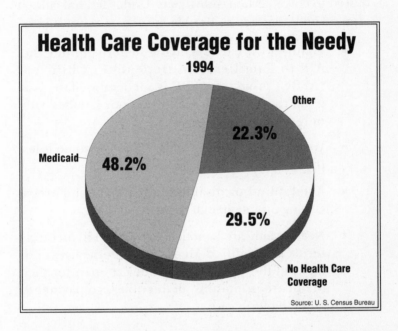

Health Care Coverage for the Needy
1994

Other 22.3%

Medicaid 48.2%

29.5%

No Health Care Coverage

Source: U. S. Census Bureau

Every needy American does not necessarily qualify for Medicaid. To receive Medicaid benefits individuals or families must first qualify for coverage under certain categories or needs. Over the years, Medicaid has been expanded to cover people with various needs. Appendix C indicates the different categories of eligibility that have been added.

Medicaid is a means-tested program, for people who earn less than a certain level of income or whose assets are less than a specified amount of money. The minimum amount of money to qualify for Medicaid varies by state. This is different than Medicare, which for the most part is a benefit received when citizens turn 65.

Even though the federal government allows states to operate their own Medicaid programs, every state is required to cover certain individuals. Under federal rules it is mandatory that states offer Medicaid to these groups:

- Families who are receiving benefits under the Aid to Families with Dependent Children (AFDC) program. AFDC is a federal welfare program that pays cash mainly to poor families with only one parent.

- Women and children whose family income is less than 133% of the poverty level.

- Aged, blind or disabled individuals who are receiving Supplemental Security Income.

- Needy Medicare beneficiaries, known in Medicaid terms as Qualified Medicare Beneficiaries. For many of these individuals, Medicaid pays for their Medicare premiums, deductibles, co-payments, and long-term care.

In addition to these Medicaid beneficiaries, each state is allowed to determine classes of other needy individuals who can receive benefits. For example, most states offer Medicaid to "medically needy" people who cannot afford insurance or pay their medical bills. These are usually individuals who do not fall under any of the categories above, but who have had their financial resources devastated by large medical expenses.

States also have the option to cover individuals who need long-term care such as nursing home care or institutional care. Almost every state offers this coverage. For the people who need this care, each state has different guidelines as to who is covered and what type of care is covered.

DIFFERENT PEOPLE, DIFFERENT NEEDS

Medicaid is a much different program than Medicare. Both programs are suffering from rising costs in the health care industry. Medicaid was created to cover a different portion of the population that requires different types of health care.

The charts below show who is covered by Medicaid and how Medicaid funds are spent. Clearly, some age groups are more expensive to care for than others.

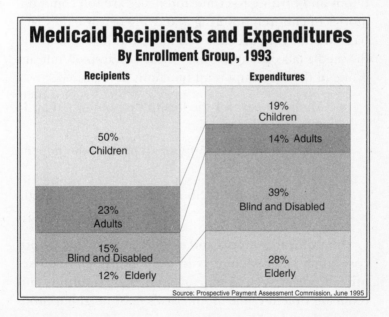

Medicaid Recipients and Expenditures
By Enrollment Group, 1993

Recipients / Expenditures

50% Children
23% Adults
15% Blind and Disabled
12% Elderly

19% Children
14% Adults
39% Blind and Disabled
28% Elderly

Source: Prospective Payment Assessment Commission, June 1995

INTENSIVE CARE

Virtually all of the expenditures associated with the blind and disabled and the elderly are for long-term care in nursing homes and other institutions.

Caring for children who need immunization shots is relatively inexpensive compared to the nursing home care described above. Increased costs are just a part of the natural process of aging.

Because Medicaid covers people of all ages, the program faces a variety of challenges. The discussion below will illustrate the diverse coverage of the Medicaid program.

CHILDREN

Poverty has its most dramatic effect on children. The horror stories of children growing up in poor neighborhoods and turning to crime and drugs are too common. Stories of children suffering and dying because they lack basic health care are also common, not just something the media talks about. Caring for the children of America is one of the most important functions of Medicaid.

- Medicaid pays for the health care of more than 16 million children.

- Children make up 50% of all people who depend on Medicaid.

- Children only use about 15% of the total Medicaid funds.

Immunization shots and periodic check-ups do not cost much and save money in the long run. Of course, other reforms such as improving living conditions and reducing violent crime in America's poor neighborhoods can cut down on Medicaid costs.

MEDICAID: THE LAST SAFETY NET

In the meantime, reforming Medicaid must include getting more children the health care they need. This is one reform that should not be difficult. Leadership is needed to make certain the system operates efficiently, which it is not doing right now.

For example, in May 1995 the Centers for Disease Control held a "National Immunization Conference" in Beverly Hills that cost more than $1 million. For this amount of money 13,500 children under the age of one year could have been given their immunization shots. Using this $1 million for action instead of talk would have benefited 13,500 children. Waste like this can be solved with pure common sense.

ADULTS

Adults, other than the elderly and disabled, account for nearly a quarter of Medicaid recipients. How adults qualify for Medicaid and the care they need is varied. Some adults might qualify for Medicaid because they are unemployed and others might qualify because they are blind or disabled. The health care needs of each adult are also very different.

Perhaps the most important group of adults that Medicaid covers is pregnant women. Caring for women while they are pregnant is crucial to having healthy babies. Because many pregnant women in the United States do not get the quality of care they need, the United States has one of the highest infant mortality rates in the industrialized world. Medicaid can make a difference in solving this problem because Medicaid pays for approximately one-third of all births in the United States.

Improving care for people such as pregnant women will help save costs in the long run. If women are healthier they will have healthier babies. Healthy babies then become healthy children, who have a better chance of becoming healthy and productive adults. So a few extra dollars spent on a pregnant woman may result in less health care costs in the future. Again, this is a common sense reform.

Caring for pregnant women and other adults does not make up a large portion of Medicaid spending. Most of the basic tests and procedures that adults need are usually not expensive. The long-term care and major illnesses that require most of the money Medicaid spends are attributable to senior citizens and disabled recipients.

SENIOR CITIZENS AND THE DISABLED

The reason senior citizens and the disabled are grouped together is because many of their health care needs are similar. Many senior and disabled Americans require long-term care. Even though *Medicare* pays for a majority of the medical costs for seniors, it does not pay for long-term care like nursing homes. Many seniors also cannot afford to pay the premiums and co-payments required by Medicare.

FOR ABOUT THREE MILLION SENIOR CITIZENS, MEDICAID PAYS THE PREMIUMS, DEDUCTIBLES AND OTHER PAYMENTS THAT MEDICARE DOES NOT COVER.

Many disabled and blind individuals also do not have sufficient income to pay for their own health care. For these people, Medicaid is an important program that they depend on during their entire lifetimes. Caring for a paralyzed person is expensive, but if this person has no insurance or the insurance runs out, who is going to pay for the care? Medicaid is often the only solution.

MEDICAID: THE LAST SAFETY NET

As the charts on page 131 illustrate, senior citizens and the disabled account for a little more than 25% of all Medicaid recipients. However, they account for about 67% of all Medicaid expenditures. The major reason for the high costs are the high demand for services and the expensive nature of long-term care. Nursing homes account for a large portion of these costs.

- **Nursing homes receive almost half their income from Medicaid.**

- **Nursing homes cost an average of $38,000 a year.**

Even though nursing home costs may seem high, the real problem is the average length of stay. An aging population will require even more money from the government for long-term care. Before this happens, the health care system must be reformed to address this important question: Who will pay for long-term care?

Many disabled people do not have the option of earning or saving money to pay for their care. In these circumstances the government has a responsibility to offer aid. It will be difficult for the federal government to continue paying for the full cost of nursing home care for a growing senior population. The people who can afford to pay for their own long-term care should not rely on the government to pay their bill.

One of the most expensive abuses of Medicaid comes from people hiding their assets in order to get Medicaid to pay for their nursing home care. In many states senior citizens with assets of less than $2,000 can get their nursing home care paid for by Medicaid. As a result, many seniors *shelter* their assets to become eligible for Medicaid.

For example, some senior citizens invest most of their cash, but put aside enough to pay for one year in a first class nursing home that can cost more than $50,000 a year. After a year this person claims that he or she has less than $2,000 in assets. Medicaid will then pay to keep him or her in this same expensive nursing home. This person can actually have hundreds of thousands of dollars legally invested while the government pays for the long-term care.

The worst part about this abuse of the system is that it is perfectly legal. Some lawyers make a living telling seniors how they can get the government to pay for this costly care. If the government is going to get control of Medicaid costs, it must stop people from taking advantage of loopholes in the law.

RISING COSTS

Medicaid spending is rising for many of the same reasons overall health care spending is rising. Because Medicaid is an integral part of the American health care system of hospitals, doctors and other providers, it is a contributor to and victim of higher costs. Like Medicare reform, controlling costs will be the main goal of Medicaid reform.

For Medicaid, a major force behind increased spending has been the system the federal government uses to pay the states. Federal spending on Medicaid is determined by a formula based on the per capita income for each state. THE FEDERAL GOVERNMENT WILL PAY BETWEEN 50% AND 83% OF MEDICAID COSTS FOR A STATE DEPENDING ON THE AVERAGE WEALTH OF ITS RESIDENTS.

MEDICAID: THE LAST SAFETY NET

States such as New York that have a higher average income per person get a smaller share of federal money than poorer states such as Mississippi. In 1993, New York received 50 cents from the federal government for every dollar it spent on Medicaid. The same year Mississippi received about 75 cents from the federal treasury for every dollar it spent on Medicaid.

This system has many flaws. **THE BIGGEST PROBLEM WITH THE CURRENT PAYMENT SYSTEM IS THAT THE MORE MONEY EACH STATE SPENDS, THE MORE MONEY IT WILL GET FROM THE FEDERAL GOVERNMENT.** Many state governments have even figured out how to get the federal government to pay more money without the state having to pay more money.

DISPROPORTIONATE ABUSE

The most frequent way states increase their share of federal funding is by abusing a system that assists hospitals that treat a high proportion of Medicaid patients. These hospitals are called *disproportionate share hospitals* (DSHs). Even though there are a few federal guidelines, state governments have the power to choose which hospitals can qualify for this aid. Under the current law, any hospital is eligible if more than 1% of the total days patients spend in the hospital are paid by Medicaid.

Aiding hospitals that treat a disproportionate amount of Medicaid recipients is a decent idea that has been abused. Some states have not only figured out how to increase their DSH payments, but they are not using this Medicaid money for health care. Here is a hypothetical example of how a state with a federal matching rate of 50% can abuse the DSH program:

1. A hospital pays a tax of $30 million to the state.
2. The state then pays the hospital a DSH payment of $40 million.
3. The state then reports to the federal government that it has spent $40 million on this DSH hospital.
4. The federal government will pay the state $20 million because the matching rate for this state is 50%.

The result is that the hospital paid $30 million, but received $40 million back for a gain of $10 million. The state government collected $30 million from the hospital and $20 million from the federal government for a total of $50 million. However, the state only pays the hospital $40 million, so the state keeps $10 million. This $10 million then becomes part of the state's general revenue and can be used for whatever the state wants from salaries to road construction.

So the state and hospital both make a profit of $10 million while the federal government loses $20 million. Remember, this is only one hospital and the matching rate was the minimum of 50%. This is a very profitable game for states. This practice has become so prevalent and well known that when states try to attract more federal funds for other programs by using similar tactics, it is called "Medicaiding."

Accounting tricks like this are a major reason why Medicaid costs have been rising. As the chart on page 139 shows, **FEDERAL DSH PAYMENTS GREW 2,500% FROM $400 MILLION TO $10.1 BILLION BETWEEN 1989 AND 1992.** Obviously, this extraordinary growth was a major contributor to the overall growth rate of Medicaid. In 1991, Congress passed legislation to address this problem. This legislation banned many of the accounting gimmicks states used, capped how much states can tax health care providers, and limited state DSH payments at no more than 12% of all Medicaid expenditures.

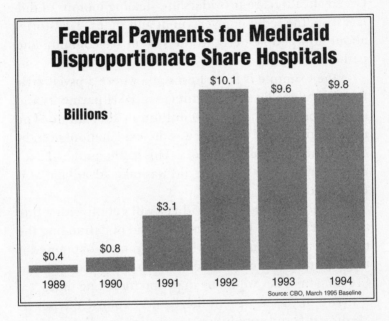

Federal Payments for Medicaid Disproportionate Share Hospitals

Billions

1989	$0.4
1990	$0.8
1991	$3.1
1992	$10.1
1993	$9.6
1994	$9.8

Source: CBO, March 1995 Baseline

This was another patchwork solution from Washington. The DSH payment system needs many more reforms. Placing a limit on DSH payments does not stop states from abusing the system, it just makes it less profitable. As part of the reform process the DSH system must be studied from the bottom to the top. RURAL HOSPITALS AND LARGE PUBLIC HOSPITALS THAT TREAT A HIGH PERCENTAGE OF MEDICAID RECIPIENTS SHOULD BE THE ONES BENEFITING FROM DSH PAYMENTS, NOT STATE GOVERNMENTS.

INTENSIVE CARE

THE FRAUD BUSINESS

While states are abusing the Medicaid system, many people are making millions of dollars more through fraud. Greedy health care providers are stealing billions of dollars from the federal government and states. The stories about how people defraud the system are common and pathetic.

One example is from Louisiana where a psychiatric hospital allegedly took advantage of DSH payments and made a profit of nearly $10 million in 1993 alone. The most tragic part of the story was the explanation given by one of the hospital's directors. This is the quote: "That's the American way — all we did was take advantage of it (Medicaid)."

Chances are these individuals will get off with a fine and perhaps some prison time. Instead of defrauding the taxpayers of $10 million, what would have happened if these same people had broken into a bank and stolen $10 million? They would be in prison for a long time.

One of the most extensive and expensive types of Medicaid fraud involves prescription medicine. This swindle involves so-called "pill mills." Sadly, the process includes doctors, pharmacists and patients. First, doctors or clinics give Medicaid recipients prescription drugs they do not need in exchange for their Medicaid number. The doctors or clinics then use the Medicaid number to bill Medicaid for unnecessary tests and procedures. In the meantime, the patients take their prescription drugs and sell them to a middleman, who turns around and sells the drugs back to the pharmacy for a fraction of their value.

MEDICAID: THE LAST SAFETY NET

This complex system has been very profitable for many people. In one state, the operators of one of these pill mills made over $8 million by defrauding the government. This is only one example of the type of fraud that adds billions of dollars to the cost of Medicaid. Here are a few more examples:

- A nationwide health care provider based in Illinois pleaded guilty to Medicaid fraud, and agreed to pay a $161 million fine. The company was accused of paying kickbacks to doctors and inflating billings.

- After non-emergency transportation services in Georgia quadrupled in three years, Medicaid officials decided to look into the companies that were billing Medicaid. After convicting nine companies of fraud, the state ended up saving $60 million in one year.

Stopping fraud will not be easy. Whenever the government puts up a safeguard, the criminals are already on to the next scam. More often than not, when someone is caught defrauding the government, the punishment does not seem to fit the crime. The government usually is not even able to collect the money that has been stolen.

With 56 different programs to monitor, it is difficult for the federal government to detect and track down fraud. At the state level, combating fraud is not easy because budget constraints have forced cuts in anti-fraud programs. The federal government must work with the states to design programs that prevent fraud. When fraud is detected the criminals who are stealing money from the taxpayers should be severely fined and punished, not just slapped on the wrist.

INTENSIVE CARE

MEDICAID AND THE ECONOMY

A major factor in Medicaid spending is the economy. When the American economy is doing well, more people are working. When more people are working there are fewer people who need Medicaid. On the other hand, if the nation goes into a recession, then unemployment will rise. When unemployment rises more people cannot afford health care and turn to Medicaid for help.

STUDIES DONE BY THE GENERAL ACCOUNTING OFFICE INDICATE THAT FOR EVERY 1% INCREASE IN THE UNEMPLOYMENT RATE, MEDICAID SPENDING INCREASES BY 6%. So if the unemployment rate increased by 1% in 1996, Medicaid spending would increase by $10 billion. Likewise, a 1% *decrease* in the unemployment rate would *save* $10 billion.

This is a cost factor over which Medicaid reform has little control. Of course, increased Medicaid spending is contributing to the national debt and straining state budgets. Once again, the road to reforming Medicaid returns to the budget. If these Medicaid costs continue to rise too fast, the deficit and debt will increase and the economy will suffer. A TROUBLED ECONOMY LEADS TO INCREASED UNEMPLOYMENT, WHICH RESULTS IN HIGHER MEDICAID COSTS. THE CYCLE IS VICIOUS.

SOCIETY'S CHALLENGES

There are many other reasons for the rising cost of Medicaid. Many of these reasons are politically sensitive. If Medicaid is ever going to be reformed, these issues must be discussed.

MEDICAID: THE LAST SAFETY NET

Many of these issues relate to personal responsibility. For example, if a person abuses alcohol and drugs his or her health will likely suffer. Is it fair for the people who take care of themselves and treat their bodies correctly to be required to pay for the health care of people who do not? This is an issue that goes beyond Medicaid or health care reform.

Drug users and alcoholics add to the cost of Medicaid. **THE EXACT COST IS UNKNOWN, BUT THE HEALTH CARE FINANCING ADMINISTRATION ESTIMATES THAT MEDICAID WILL SPEND ABOUT $700 MILLION IN 1995 JUST CARING FOR DRUG ABUSERS.**

There are many horror stories about the amount of money that seems to be wasted. For example, in Seattle five alcoholics had to be taken to detoxification centers more than once because they had abused their bodies to the point of danger. These trips cost the taxpayers half a million dollars. The alcoholics never had to pay a dime. Issues like this will be difficult to solve, but if Medicaid spending is to be controlled, an answer must be found.

The cost of treating smokers is another issue that is gaining attention. In February 1995, the state of Florida sued tobacco manufacturers for $1.4 billion. The state claims this is how much money Medicaid has spent to treat people with health problems related to using tobacco.

If someone smokes, should the government have to pay for his or her increased health care costs? If not, who should pay? These are difficult questions that must be discussed in the reform process. There will be no answer that is popular with everyone.

Another difficult issue to address is immigration. Most of the people who *legally* immigrate into the United

States do not contribute to the rising cost of Medicaid. These individuals usually have a job before they enter the country. They pay taxes and usually receive health care benefits from their employer.

The people who enter the United States *illegally* are a different story. In places like Southern California people from Mexico come into the United States just to receive health care. Women from Mexico travel to American emergency rooms to give birth because they know they will get the best health care the world has to offer. The federal government must decide whether it can afford to give costly health care to immigrants who illegally enter the United States.

Denying health care to these people is not the ultimate answer. It is inhumane not to care for a person in need. The answer lies beyond health care policy. It is a question of immigration policy that Washington must address. Some fair measures must be taken because the United States can barely afford to care for its own people.

Another contributor to the rising cost of Medicaid is caring for people with AIDS. Estimates by the Health Care Financing Administration indicate that in 1995 Medicaid will spend about $1.6 billion on AIDS care. Some studies show that at least 40% of the people that have the HIV virus will eventually become a Medicaid recipient. This is a contemporary problem of huge proportions that is contributing to the cost of Medicaid.

Endless rounds of short-term reforms have ignored these issues. It is time for real reform that looks into every aspect of the system. This is the only road to real, meaningful and lasting reform.

9

Medicaid Reform: Solving the Puzzle

Updating Medicaid will be like solving a difficult and complicated puzzle. Every single piece of the program does not always seem to fit correctly with the other pieces. Medicaid cares for a variety of people with many different needs.

For these reasons some reforms will be needed that are aimed only at specific parts of Medicaid. Other reforms will address problems with the entire Medicaid program. Changes to the entire health care industry will also be needed. A diverse program demands diverse solutions.

Possibilities for modernizing the entire health care system will obviously have a tremendous impact on the Medicaid program. Managed care and Medical Savings Accounts are two of the most talked about possibilities for system-wide reform. Managed care will be discussed briefly in this chapter and in more detail in Chapter 10. Medical Savings Accounts will be the topic of Chapter 11.

INTENSIVE CARE

Experts in public policy and in the health care industry propose a variety of reform ideas that might work for the Medicaid program. Each one of these ideas deserves to be studied and analyzed. If a reform proposal makes sense, it first should be tested on a limited basis.

Only by pilot testing many common sense reforms will their true benefits and problems become known. The Medicaid system is a great laboratory. With 56 different programs, various reform proposals can be tested and closely scrutinized at the same time.

The ideas outlined in this chapter are possible solutions that are specific to Medicaid. By no means does this list include every available alternative. Any reasonable reform proposal should be given consideration.

FAIR PAY

One of the first and easiest reforms Medicaid can accomplish is making the disproportionate share hospital (DSH) payment system fair. As Chapter 8 explained, this system has grown out of control because it has been abused.

This reform should be relatively simple. DSH payments were created to aid hospitals that treat a large number of needy patients. Because these hospitals often incur higher costs when treating low-income individuals, the federal government offers these hospitals extra aid. State governments have found ways to take advantage of this system. Rather than using their talents to develop meaningful solutions to health care problems, state governments have been devising methods to extract money from the federal government.

MEDICAID REFORM: SOLVING THE PUZZLE

THE GROWTH OF DSH PAYMENTS FROM $400 MILLION IN 1989 TO $10.1 BILLION IN 1992 IS PROOF ENOUGH THAT THIS SYSTEM HAS BEEN ABUSED. The federal government gave states too much leeway in deciding which hospitals can receive DSH payments. Congress has recently tried to curb this abuse, but curbing the abuse is not enough. The practice must be stopped completely.

The hospitals that are actually treating a disproportionate share of needy Americans should be the ones getting this money. These hospitals are doing a service to the nation, and they deserve some extra funding.

Before beginning to reform other parts of the system, waste, fraud, and abuse must be eliminated. DSH payments were never meant to be used by the states as part of their general funds. These are health care dollars that should be spent on health care. At a time when Medicaid costs are rising rapidly, every dollar makes a difference.

CARING FOR COMMUNITIES

Before Medicaid took over as the dominant provider of health care for needy Americans, charity hospitals cared for millions of people in rural areas and cities. When Medicaid was formed, the government soon became the main health care payer for the needy.

Medicaid helps fund over 600 urban hospitals and over 2,000 rural clinics. These community health facilities benefit millions of Americans. They serve as teaching and research centers that are the backbone of the nation's health care system.

Community health centers offer important services in poor areas. In many places, they are the only source of health care. These facilities also have been able to provide care that is relatively inexpensive. For example, a study of six urban health centers in New York revealed that it cost 41% less to care for patients in these urban health centers than in alternative health care facilities.

Some of these rural and urban facilities are serving the needs of their communities at a reasonable price. Expanding their use might be one way for Medicaid to improve quality and access while controlling costs.

In many large cities, these community centers are major hospitals. One reform idea is to build smaller clinics around these cities. These clinics would offer Medicaid recipients basic and primary care.

The advantage is that many patients would no longer have to rely on busy trauma centers for their minor health care needs. Smaller clinics located near the patients' homes would be able to serve Medicaid recipients more quickly and for less money. The larger hospitals would benefit because they would not have to care for minor ailments. All their energy and resources could be directed toward complex emergency work.

Finding the money and staff to operate community centers will be difficult. In rural areas, finding qualified doctors is a common problem. A major obstacle for cities and rural areas is paying the construction and operating costs of these clinics.

In some areas private companies are building their own community clinics. Private companies, such as managed care organizations, are teaming up with large hospitals and offering preventive and primary care to Medicaid recipients.

This relationship can benefit everyone involved. Hospital trauma centers do not have to worry about non-emergency care. Patients know they can go to their community clinic and not wait in line all day. Plus, these clinics are much more personal, allowing patients to build a relationship with their doctors. If operated correctly, private companies can actually make a profit from these clinics while Medicaid saves money.

INSURING THE NEEDY

Under the current Medicaid system, the federal government serves as the health care insurer for most of the 33 million people who rely on the program. Because it is financed by the American taxpayers, Medicaid is not a typical insurance company.

A proposed alternative to this system is to change the role of the government from an insurer to a purchaser of insurance. This *voucher* system would allow Medicaid recipients to purchase their own health care plans with federal money.

Every year needy Americans who qualify for Medicaid would be given a voucher worth a certain amount of money. The value of each voucher would be enough to purchase private insurance or a managed care plan that covers their health care needs. In most states, that amount would most likely be $3,000 to $4,000 for a family of three.

This voucher would enable Medicaid recipients to purchase a health care plan that is suitable for them. People in different areas have special needs. Vouchers would allow them to shop around for a policy that offers the best care and benefits.

Insurers would compete for the vouchers by offering a variety of benefits and different levels of deductibles and co-payments. In theory, this competitive marketplace would drive down costs and save the government money.

One potential problem of this voucher system is that federal money will go to insurance companies and not directly to public hospitals. Many of the largest hospitals in the nation serve as research and teaching centers. These hospitals rely on Medicaid patients for a large part of their income.

Medicaid recipients are likely to use their vouchers to purchase managed care plans. Because many managed care organizations own hospitals and employ doctors, public hospitals and clinics would lose a large patient base and millions of dollars from Medicaid.

This is another example of the complexity of the Medicaid puzzle. Vouchers may save money, but threaten the public health care system. When one piece of the puzzle starts to fit, another piece pops out.

Vouchers may drastically transform the current Medicaid system by shifting more patients into the hands of private care. Instead of changing the system as a whole, some reform options are based on changing the financing and administration of Medicaid. The main goal of these reforms would be to save money without changing the quality of and access to care.

BLOCK GRANTS

An expensive problem with the current system is the matching funds system that is used to pay for Medicaid. Chapter 8 discussed the situation of the states that spend more money on Medicaid than other states. These higher-spending states receive even more money from the federal government.

MEDICAID REFORM: SOLVING THE PUZZLE

One way to solve this problem is to give states block grants for Medicaid. Under this system each state would receive a predetermined amount of money annually from the federal government. Most likely a block grant would be slightly less than the amount each state now receives. In return for less money, the federal government gives states more control to run their own programs.

For example, in 1993 Illinois spent about $5 billion on Medicaid. Because the state's federal matching rate is 50%, Illinois received about $2.5 billion from the federal government. Under a block grant, Illinois would be given a set amount such as $2.2 billion. The federal government would save about $300 million and in return Illinois would have more control over its Medicaid program.

A major question about block grants is how the government would be able to handle them during economic recessions. Medicaid enrollment is affected by the unemployment rate. Because block grants set a specific federal spending level, the system cannot compensate for increased Medicaid beneficiaries.

If a state is suffering from a recession, unemployment will rise and the state's tax revenue will suffer. If this happened today, the federal government is able to pick up part of the increased costs for the state. Block grants may not be able to compensate for changing economic conditions.

To help compensate for higher program costs when the economy is in trouble, Congress could establish an emergency fund. This fund would put away money to pay for Medicaid costs when tax revenue is less than expected. The problem is that under the accounting practices of the federal government this fund would most likely become another trust fund.

INTENSIVE CARE

Determining how much each state should receive under a block grant program will be a bitter debate. Under the current system states spend varying amounts on Medicaid recipients. In 1993 Indiana spent an average of more than $1,900 on each child receiving Medicaid. The same year Alabama spent less than $600 per child on Medicaid.

Another problem that would need to be addressed is how to compensate states that have high growth rates. States such as Florida are growing much faster than most other states. As a result, over a period of time Florida would require more money.

With 56 different Medicaid programs in operation, forming a block grant system that is fair to the states and meets the needs of the participants will be difficult.

FEDERAL CONTROL

Another approach to restructuring Medicaid is to give the federal government full control over the program. Under such a program, the federal government would have complete responsibility for the financing and administration of Medicaid.

Supporters of this idea believe that placing the control of Medicaid into federal hands will help control medical costs. Operating a single program instead of 56 different programs, the federal government may be able to design one system that operates more efficiently.

Medicaid beneficiaries across the country could get equal treatment because the federal government would set standard benefits and eligibility requirements. Currently, there is a wide variation of benefits and eligibility among states. As a result, many Medicaid beneficiaries move, or *migrate*, to states that give more generous benefits.

The downside of the federal government taking control of the entire Medicaid program is that another bureaucracy might be the end result. In this case the government is only trading one set of problems for another set. The federal government also cannot afford to run Medicaid by itself. Somehow states would have to contribute to the cost.

SPLITTING RESPONSIBILITIES

Splitting Medicaid into two distinct programs run by different levels of the government is another possible reform. One idea is to let the federal government be responsible for acute and primary care and let the states be responsible for long-term care. Other proposals suggest just the opposite.

Because acute and primary care and long-term care are very different, separating the two into different programs may improve Medicaid in many ways. Proponents of this split believe it will bring more attention to the needs of Medicaid recipients. Quality may improve and costs decline if each type of care is operated separately.

Which level of government should operate which type of care would be a controversial topic. Since long-term care is so expensive, states and the federal government will claim the other should pay for this portion of Medicaid. Once again the cost factor becomes the final test.

Restructuring responsibilities will alter the administration and payment of Medicaid. It does not necessarily mean that rising costs can be controlled. Even if Medicaid is restructured, other reforms will still be needed. Perhaps the most well known of these reforms is managed care.

MANAGING MEDICAID

Within the last decade a growing number of Medicaid recipients have been moved into managed care plans. The chart on page 155 shows the increasing use of this option by the Medicaid program. In 1994 nearly eight million Medicaid recipients were enrolled in managed care plans.

There are two basic ideas behind using managed care plans for Medicaid recipients. First, managed care plans are purchased for a set fee. All costs incurred by a patient are covered in full for the term of the policy. This can limit how much money the government has to spend on managed care patients because the only cost Medicaid must cover is the insurance premium for the plan.

The second potential benefit is that managed care plans have primary doctors that oversee a patient's health care. For Medicaid recipients this is an added benefit because they can get preventive and acute care when they need it.

Unlike many other proposed reforms, managed care is currently being tested by numerous states. Many other states are also considering greater use of managed care plans.

For a state to overhaul its Medicaid program to include managed care coverage requires a waiver from the Health Care Financing Administration (HCFA). As of early 1995, waivers had been approved for Florida,

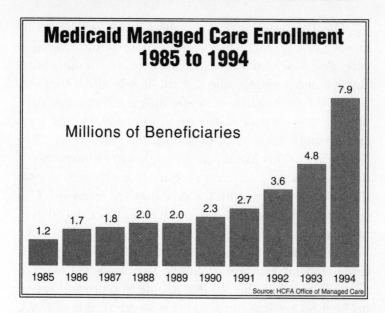

Medicaid Managed Care Enrollment 1985 to 1994

Millions of Beneficiaries

1985	1986	1987	1988	1989	1990	1991	1992	1993	1994
1.2	1.7	1.8	2.0	2.0	2.3	2.7	3.6	4.8	7.9

Source: HCFA Office of Managed Care

Hawaii, Kentucky, Ohio, Oregon, Rhode Island and Tennessee. At least fifteen other states have either already applied or are considering applying for the waiver.

The main purpose of these waivers is to get more people into managed care, which will supposedly save money. These savings will be directed towards expanding coverage to new recipients.

Each waiver lasts for five years. Over that five-year period the federal government may increase its funding if the program is enrolling new recipients. At the end of that five years, HCFA will cut back funding for the recipients that have been added. In theory, after five years the savings from moving people into managed care should be enough to offset the cost of expanding coverage.

Unlike many other reforms that are being discussed, managed care is already being used to a large extent. The most ambitious program began in 1994 in Tennessee.

INTENSIVE CARE

The Tennessee program, called TennCare, began by moving nearly 900,00 Medicaid recipients into managed care. The next step was to provide coverage to more than 400,000 needy people who did not have health insurance.

TennCare consists of twelve different managed care organizations that provide care to all enrollees. The average annual payment per enrollee is about $1,500. TennCare allows Medicaid recipients to choose one of the twelve plans. Every year recipients can change plans if they are not pleased with the care they are receiving. This competition is designed to create a market that drives prices down while improving quality.

TennCare started on January 1, 1994, so it is premature to label it a success or failure. In only its first year the program enrolled the 400,000 people who previously had no health care insurance. This is an admirable success. The problem is that during the first year, the program ran a $99 million deficit.

Managed care and some of the reforms that have been mentioned all have their potential benefits and problems. Each one deserves to be reviewed closely. However, none of these reforms by themselves will get health care costs under control. Other reforms are needed that will reform Medicaid, Medicare, and every other part of the American health care system.

Two reforms that are being discussed in Washington, D.C. and state capitals across the nation are a variety of different managed care plans and Medical Savings Accounts. These two reforms will be important pieces in the entire health care puzzle.

10

Managed Health Care

No discussion of health care today is complete without an understanding of the area of the health care industry known as *managed care.* Chapters 7 and 9 discussed various reform proposals that included this option. To better understand how managed care works requires a separate chapter.

The chart on page 158 indicates that during the past decade the number of people enrolled in the most well-known type of managed care plan — health maintenance organizations — has risen from 19 million in 1985 to 41 million in 1992. Even though they recently have been gaining recognition and popularity, managed care plans have been in existence for decades.

As early as the 1940s managed care was available in California, Washington, Oregon and New York. Back then, managed care consisted of health maintenance organizations (HMOs). HMOs combined the insurer and health care provider into one. The HMO would hire its own doctors, and patients were allowed to only visit these doctors.

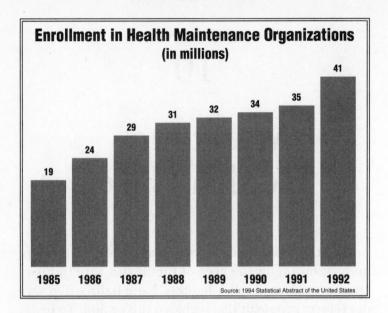

Enrollment in Health Maintenance Organizations
(in millions)

Year	Enrollment
1985	19
1986	24
1987	29
1988	31
1989	32
1990	34
1991	35
1992	41

Source: 1994 Statistical Abstract of the United States

Over the years managed care has expanded and changed with the times. Today, managed care usually refers to any insurance or health care plan that involves a primary care doctor that oversees, or manages, a patient's care. The goal of a managed care plan is to seek the best health care value.

Patients enrolled in a managed care plan agree to see doctors that are either employed by or under contract to the managed care organization. For example, HMO patients pay a set fee and most of their health care needs are met by the organization. There usually are no additional costs for the patient. Because patients pay all their costs up front, HMOs are sometimes referred to as prepaid plans.

In a traditional health care plan — called an indemnity plan — patients can visit any doctor they choose. The patient then pays the bill and a percentage of the bill —

usually about 80% — is reimbursed by their insurance company.

Today, it is difficult to tell the difference between a traditional plan and a modern managed care plan. Perhaps the easiest way to distinguish a managed care plan from a traditional plan is by whether or not there is a primary care doctor. A patient in a managed care plan must first go to his or her primary care doctor, who then determines the patient's health care needs. For example, if a patient is suffering from back pain, he or she must go to their primary care doctor first. This doctor will then determine which specialist the patient should see.

Primary care doctors are intended to keep patients from overusing the health care system. There are opposing viewpoints as to the effectiveness of this process. Critics refer to the primary doctors as *gatekeepers*, claiming they keep patients away from the care they need. Supporters say that the primary care doctor is just the modern version of the trusted family doctor.

Managed care today cannot always be defined according to the presence of a family doctor. As society and the health care profession have become more complex, so has the definition of managed care.

ABCs OF HEALTH CARE

When any health care professional begins talking about the various types of health care plans now available, it sounds as if someone is just reciting the alphabet in some random order. The health care industry is filled with acronyms for different plans.

INTENSIVE CARE

People in the health care industry are always talking about HMOs, FFS, IPAs, POSs, PPOs and other types of service that seem to require three initials.

To be able to understand the options that many health insurers offer, it helps to know what each of these acronyms means.

- **HEALTH MAINTENANCE ORGANIZATIONS (HMOs)** combine insurance and health care into one. HMOs sell policies and also provide health care, which allows them to better control costs. Patients, known as members, pay a fixed fee that covers all their medical costs. Members agree to only go to doctors and hospitals that are part of the HMO.

- **FEE FOR SERVICE (FFS)** is a traditional type of health care insurance where the insurance companies pay health care providers according to the services that are provided. Usually, the plan includes a deductible and a co-payment.

- **INDIVIDUAL PRACTICE ASSOCIATIONS (IPAs)** are a type of HMO that contracts with an association of private doctors. The HMO contracts with the IPA, and then the IPA in turn contracts with a network of doctors.

- **POINT OF SERVICE (POS)** plans are similar to HMOs, but allow patients to choose doctors outside of the plan. However, if patients do go outside the plan's network, they are required to pay a larger co-payment, or portion of their doctor's bill.

MANAGED HEALTH CARE

- **PREFERRED PROVIDER ORGANIZATIONS (PPOs)** contract with selected doctors and hospitals instead of hiring their own doctors and owning their own hospitals. If patients go to these providers the PPO will pay most of the costs. If the patient goes outside of this network the patient's costs will be higher.

Confused? Many of these different plans such as PPOs, IPOs and FFS plans are similar. A few minor differences give them different names. In the past there was a clear difference between a traditional plan and a managed care plan. That difference is now blurred.

One example of a hybrid between a managed care plan and a traditional plan is a *managed indemnity plan*. Like a normal indemnity plan, patients with this type of coverage can go to any provider. However, a third party reviews all the bills and determines whether or not they are acceptable. This can be considered a managed care plan because of the presence of this third party.

CONTROLLING COSTS

One of the major goals of managed care plans is to control the cost of health care. Because they either hire their own providers or contract with outside providers, managed care organizations limit patients to certain doctors and hospitals.

If an HMO employs its own doctors and owns its own hospitals, the organization can control many of its costs. In a traditional plan, an insurer has little control over costs because they have to pay any reasonable charge from a doctor or hospital.

INTENSIVE CARE

There is evidence that managed care can save money by controlling costs. In 1994, HMO and PPO enrollment in the private sector increased by 21%. During that year, the health care costs for American businesses actually decreased by 1.1%.

It is unknown whether this savings is a result of managed care or an industry-wide change in health care costs. While managed care organizations claim they are responsible for declining costs, skeptics say that these organizations may be cutting back on health care services to save money and increase profits.

THE PROFIT MOTIVE

The debate over whether or not managed care organizations place profit over quality of care will probably never be settled. Supporters are armed with evidence that managed care plans control health care spending, making quality health care affordable. Skeptics claim that in order to make a profit managed care organizations must either cut spending or raise revenues.

Managed care is often blamed for cutting costs at the expense of necessary care. For example, some HMOs are cutting their hospital costs by discharging patients earlier than normal. Under some plans, women are being sent home from the hospital less than 12 hours after giving birth.

Because many HMOs are run as for-profit businesses, this profit motive is becoming a prominent topic in the health care community. In 1994, the CEOs of some of the largest for-profit HMOs received an average of $7 million *each* in compensation for the year.

MANAGED HEALTH CARE

The profit motive in managed care is not necessarily a problem. It can also force competing plans to improve their care in order to attract and keep customers. In effect, the marketplace is at work.

It is too early to determine whether the advantages of managed care outweigh the disadvantages, or vice-versa. The American health care system has undergone a fundamental change with health care providers operating as a big business. The complete effect of this change is not yet known.

Medicare and Medicaid recipients should be given the option to select from a variety of health care plans. This is the only way the true benefits and problems with managed care will become known. If managed care works, people will use it. If not, the market will force the plans to change.

MANAGED CARE, MEDICARE AND MEDICAID

Increasing the use of managed care in the Medicare and Medicaid programs is frequently mentioned as a possible solution to controlling the rising costs threatening these programs. The chart on page 164 shows that managed plans are much more popular in the private sector than in Medicare and Medicaid.

Approximately 15% of the Medicaid population is now enrolled in managed care plans. For many Medicaid recipients, managed care allows the patient to see the same primary doctor every time and increases access to preventive care. Supporters say this gives Medicaid recipients a sense of security knowing they can get care when they need it. Others disagree.

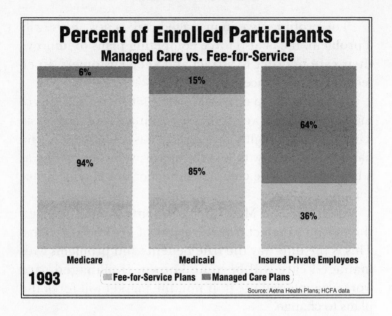

Percent of Enrolled Participants
Managed Care vs. Fee-for-Service

6%

15%

64%

94%

85%

36%

Medicare   Medicaid   Insured Private Employees

1993   ▪ Fee-for-Service Plans ▪ Managed Care Plans

Source: Aetna Health Plans; HCFA data

One of the claims critics have against giving Medicaid recipients HMO coverage, is that HMOs do not cut down on abuse. Primary doctors can limit a patient's care to an extent. However, patients are not limited to how often they may visit their primary doctor.

While Medicaid has moved about 15% of its recipients into managed care, only about 6% of Medicare beneficiaries are enrolled in managed care plans. Managed care plans may benefit senior citizens because the plans limit out-of-pocket costs. In addition, some managed care plans will pay for benefits such as eyeglasses and prescription drugs that Medicare does not cover. Whether the combination of managed care and Medicare actually saves money is disputable.

Medicare currently pays managed care plans 95% of the average annual cost of caring for a beneficiary. For the sake of making the math easier, assume that Medicare spends $1,000 on the average beneficiary every year. Medicare would pay $950 to purchase an HMO plan. The advantage would be that the beneficiary would have few, if any, out-of-pocket costs. Additionally, the government would save $50.

Medicare pays managed care organizations according to the *average* cost per beneficiary. Healthier beneficiaries cost less than the average. Assume that a relatively healthy 65-year-old beneficiary only costs Medicare an average of $600 a year. Medicare will still pay an HMO $950. The result is that Medicare actually loses $350 for that year by buying a managed care plan.

For this reason, some HMOs have been accused of only signing up healthy beneficiaries — a practice called skimming. Reports of HMO marketing representatives attending square dance festivals and swim meets for senior citizens are not uncommon. It is not fair to say every HMO engages in this practice. *In fact, some studies show that Medicare patients in managed care have the same health characteristics as the average population.*

WITHHOLDING JUDGMENT

As proven by the number of Americans who are enrolled in managed care plans, this type of health care coverage is obviously popular in the private sector. Various studies show that employees enrolled in these plans are generally pleased with the service and care they receive.

However, the most important question about managed care has yet to be answered: **DOES MANAGED CARE GET HEALTH CARE COSTS UNDER CONTROL WHILE MAINTAINING QUALITY? IT IS STILL TOO EARLY TO TELL.**

INTENSIVE CARE

As previously mentioned, HMOs and similar plans have been around for decades, but only recently has their popularity become widespread. Supporters of managed care have anecdotal evidence and surveys that their plans cost employers less and offer employees quality care. Critics have their own horror stories about poor quality of care and how managed care is just as expensive as traditional plans.

Basically, there is no absolute answer to whether or not managed care saves money and maintains or improves quality. As a U.S. General Accounting Office study stated:

> *A definitive evaluation of managed care does not exist because of a lack of clear definition, difficulty in obtaining data, the high cost of conducting an evaluation, and the constantly changing structure of managed care.*

So, can managed care help control Medicare and Medicaid costs? The only way to ever find out is to give Medicare and Medicaid recipients the option to choose the type of plan they prefer.

Patients — the consumers — will determine if managed care meets their needs. Our elected leaders will determine what the government can afford. Until it is put to the test and studied closely, we will not know how managed care can help in reforming Medicare and Medicaid.

11

Medical
Savings Accounts

One of the greatest attributes of the American people is our creativity. Throughout our history from Ben Franklin to the Wright Brothers to the men and women who are making computers smaller and faster every day, Americans have discovered ingenious ways to improve society.

In the challenge to reform the American health care system, we need creative people to think beyond the existing options. Policy architects in Washington need to take creativity lessons. If Thomas Edison can invent the light bulb, then surely some new health care reform solutions can be designed. It will take hard work and determination.

One idea for health care reform is called a Medical Savings Account (MSA), which is also known as a MediSave account or Medical IRA account. The father of this idea is Dr. John Goodman of the National Center for Policy Analysis. Most of the information in this chapter is a result of the work of Dr. Goodman and his associates.

They have spent years developing this idea. This chapter describes their plan.

Medical Savings Accounts alone will not solve the problems with Medicare, Medicaid and the entire health care system. However, it is one idea that should be tried in the marketplace. Policy makers will argue about the advantages and disadvantages of ideas like this, but until they are tested under real life conditions we will not know the true results.

HOW DO MSAs WORK?

Assume that you are the head of a typical American family. You have a spouse and two children. Every year your employer spends about $5,000 to purchase a traditional health care insurance policy that covers your entire family.

Under this policy, assume that your deductible would be $500 per family member. This means that you must pay the first $500 worth of health care costs for the year for each family member. After this $500 deductible has been met, you must pay 20% of all health care expenses up to $5,000. If your health care costs exceed $5,000 the insurance company will pay 100%.

Instead of purchasing this normal $5,000 policy, what would happen if your employer decided to purchase a catastrophic insurance plan that has a $3,000 deductible? The policy would be much cheaper, it would probably cost about $2,000.

Your employer would then give you the extra $3,000 that was saved. This money would be put into a special savings account for your health care needs — your Medical Savings Account. Whenever you or someone in your family needed health care, this account would be used to pay the bills. Once all $3,000 was used up, the insurance policy would pay the rest.

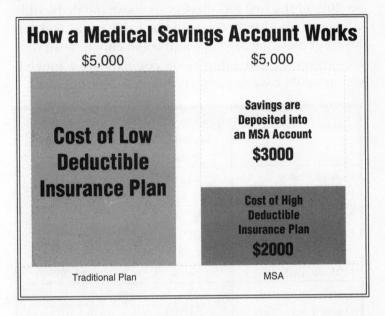

How a Medical Savings Account Works

$5,000 $5,000

Cost of Low Deductible Insurance Plan

Savings are Deposited into an MSA Account
$3000

Cost of High Deductible Insurance Plan
$2000

Traditional Plan   MSA

The above chart compares a typical low-deductible insurance plan to an MSA with a high-deductible plan. As indicated, the total spending levels are the same. However, there are some potential advantages to the MSA plan.

ADVANTAGES OF AN MSA

Compared to a traditional plan, MSAs can limit a patient's out-of-pocket costs. By the time the deductible and co-payments on a low deductible health care plan are paid, the costs could be substantial.

INTENSIVE CARE

Assume that you are an employee whose employer has decided to offer an MSA. If you had traditional health insurance with a $500 deductible and you had to pay 20% of the first $5,000 of costs above the deductible (which equals $1,000) you could be liable for $1,500. On the other hand, an MSA account could eliminate all your personal costs. The table below compares how much a person would have to pay under the two different plans.

Out-of-Pocket Costs		
	Traditional Policy	Medical Savings Account Policy
Cost of Policy	$5,000	$2,000
Deductible	$ 500	$3,000
Maximum Co-payment	$1,000 (20% of $5,000)	n/a
MSA deposit	n/a	$3,000
Total Out-of-Pocket Costs	$1,500	$ 0

Another potential advantage of MSAs is that employee's could keep any extra money that is left in the account at the end of the year. What would happen if a young couple only spends $1,500 of their $3,000 each year? If tax laws were changed, the $1,500 that is left over could be put into a tax-free account for future health care needs.

Assume that this couple put $1,500 into the account every year for ten years and invested the money. If their average return on their investment was 8% each year, this couple would have over $23,000 at the end of the 10-year period. This could be used when this couple's future medical costs rise.

MSAs AT WORK

The idea of an MSA is much more than a concept that looks good on paper. Many companies around the country are now offering this option to their employees. One of these companies is the Golden Rule Insurance Co.

Golden Rule allows their employees to choose between a traditional plan like the one shown in the table on page 170, or an MSA. In 1994, 90% of the company's workers selected the MSA option.

Under this plan, Golden Rule purchases a catastrophic plan with a $3,000 deductible. The company then deposits $2,000 into the employee's MSA, which also covers his or her family.

As a result, the most a Golden Rule employee would have to pay is $1,000. The out-of-pocket cost for the MSA policy shown in the table on page 170 would be $1,000 instead of $0. However, this is still $500 cheaper than the traditional policy.

At the end of the year, if the employee has money left is his or her account, the money can be withdrawn.

MSAs are also saving money for employers.

- In 1993, the first year Golden Rule offered MSAs, the company's **HEALTH CARE COSTS WERE 40% LOWER** than they would have been if the company had not offered the MSA option.

- *Forbes* magazine, which uses a similar type of MSA, **SAW ITS HEALTH CARE COSTS FALL 17% IN 1992 AND 12% IN 1993.**

INTENSIVE CARE

MSAs, MEDICARE & MEDICAID

Whether or not MSAs would benefit Medicare and Medicaid recipients is a subject of much debate. Critics say that MSAs will only benefit young and healthy people because they spend less on health care and can save more money. Supporters, however, say that MSAs can work for senior citizens because MSAs would limit the high out-of-pocket costs many Medicare recipients now pay.

If MSAs were offered as a Medicare option, the government would purchase a high-deductible plan and give each enrollee money for their health care account. If the deductible were $3,000 and the enrollee had $3,000 in their MSA, they would have no out-of-pockets costs.

If the deductible were $3,000 and each enrollee received $2,000, the maximum this recipient would be expected to pay would be $1,000. Under the current system, a Medicare recipient can spend much more than $1,000 on a Medigap policy alone.

For Medicaid recipients, MSAs would allow them to choose from a variety of health care providers. Today, many Medicaid recipients will wait for hours in busy emergency rooms if they have the flu. By providing MSAs to the needy, they can use their money and go to the doctors and health care facilities of their choice.

This system would also benefit health care providers. According to the Congressional Budget Office, Medicare only pays doctors and hospitals about 70% of the fees normally charged by hospitals and doctors.

By giving patients the power of the purse, Medicare recipients would be able to shop around for the best care at the most reasonable price. Also, doctors could charge fees that are fair and not have to worry about the government undercompensating them. Again, the market-place would be at work.

OVERUSED AND UNDER USED

For most patients, the cost of their health care is not a factor in choosing their providers. Third-party payers — whether it is the government in the form of Medicare and Medicaid or private health insurance companies — are receiving and paying most of the health care bills in the United States.

WHEN SOMEONE ELSE IS PAYING THE BILL, PATIENTS TEND TO BE LESS CONCERNED ABOUT THE COST OF THE SERVICE.

By giving patients control of their own health care money, the system will not be overused. Patients would not go to expensive hospital emergency rooms when they have a cold if they have to pay for it. Instead, they would go to their local doctor.

A potential problem with this system is that many people would place saving money above their health. If they knew that they could keep the MSA money if it was not spent, they might reduce their health care. This is a valid concern, especially for needy individuals such as Medicaid recipients who will be tempted to spend this extra money for other necessities.

Individuals would have to exercise common sense to know this money is reserved for their health care needs. If they spend it, they are going to have to find another way to pay their health care bills.

AT SOME POINT, PEOPLE MUST TAKE THE RESPONSIBILITY FOR THEIR OWN LIVES. The government may help, but it cannot provide for everything we want.

INTENSIVE CARE

Just as one shoe will not fit every foot, the details of how an MSA system would work would vary from program to program and state to state. Medicare would probably have different rules than Medicaid, and California different rules than Maine.

How MSAs would work on a large-scale basis cannot be known until they are pilot tested. The appropriate laws should be passed to make MSAs a viable option for employers, employees and the people who rely on the government for their health care needs. Medical Savings Accounts may not be a complete solution to reforming the entire health care system, but they may be a good start.

•   •   •

It is time for our elected leaders to bring Medicare and Medicaid in for an emergency landing. The men and women in the congressional cockpit must work as a team to save the passengers. Creativity and determination are needed to ensure that no one gets hurt.

Once safely on the ground, our 30-year-old airplane must be updated and modernized to prevent another brush with disaster. Society has drastically changed since the 1960s. Preparing the aircraft for the 21st century will take great vision, patience and understanding.

There is no question that an overhaul is needed, but it will be well worth the effort. Medicare and Medicaid have proven to be beneficial programs for millions of Americans.

Even after our plane has been updated and modernized, no one would consider putting it back in the air without extensive testing and evaluation. Test flights should be made in as many different environments as possible before passengers are allowed to board once again.

Likewise, proposals to update and improve Medicare and Medicaid should also be pilot tested in different locations. There should be no requirement that the same program must be adopted throughout the United States. What works in Miami may not work in Seattle.

Unlike its first 30 years in operation, our aircraft will undergo regularly scheduled maintenance from now on. So, too, should Medicare and Medicaid. These programs need to be dynamic. If something isn't working or if someone has a better idea, enough flexibility needs to be built into the systems so they can be changed without rewriting thousands of pages of regulations.

Making plans to update and modernize our airplane is a great first step. Actually completing the work will take time, and pilot testing the aircraft may take even more time. But once these steps are completed, we should have a reliable and cost-efficient means of travel that meets the needs of our passengers.

So, are we ready to flip on the auto-pilot and settle back in our seats? Hardly. More work remains to be done. This next job will be very difficult.

If we are successful, however, it will be the equivalent of flying in blue skies on a cloudless day.

12

Beyond Medicine to a Healthy Society

Honorable men and women place four things on a pedestal, high above everything else: their moral and ethical beliefs, their family, their nation, and their health. Caring for all four are the primary duties of loyal citizens. Succeeding at each one of these takes responsibility and sacrifice. Failing at any of these results in tragedy.

The health of every person, family and nation depends on the health of one another. America cannot prosper if her people are ill. Likewise, the American people cannot prosper if their nation is suffering.

Health transcends physical well-being. A society that is great must be strong physically, mentally, politically, and financially. These are the reasons the United States became a superpower. These attributes need strengthening.

History teaches us how this nation became great. The successes of the past must be built upon. We should learn from our failures.

INTENSIVE CARE

In the early days of this nation, agricultural communities served as the heart of a prospering and hard-working country. These were the days Thomas Jefferson wrote about. Communities were self-reliant systems. People — citizens — helped each other in times of need. Even in the cities, citizens worked together for the good of their community.

When Alexis de Tocqueville traveled the United States in the 1830s, he realized the strength of these communities. He wrote:

> *Local assemblies of citizens constitute the strength of free nations. . . . A nation may establish a system of free government, but without the spirit of municipal institutions it cannot have the spirit of liberty.*

The nation that de Tocqueville studied has changed. Around the turn of the century, America's cities began growing at remarkable rates. Jefferson's agricultural society became an industrial society.

Technology profoundly changed the lives of all Americans. Many of the families that had worked the land for their living were replaced by farm machinery. Their only option was to migrate to the cities. Between 1901 and 1910 nearly 9 million immigrants entered the United States. Most of these immigrants also moved into the cities. The American melting pot was formed.

America's growing urban centers brought new challenges. Factories replaced the fields as the place of employment. These factories were nothing like modern factories. This was the era where blood, sweat and tears were not a figure of speech; they were a fact of life.

Factories were difficult and dangerous places to work. Conditions were intolerable. Workers were often mauled and lost their arms and legs in factory accidents. Benefits such as overtime pay and workers compensation were years away. There was a legitimate need for government regulation.

Outside of work, conditions were not much better. Many families lived in spaces that by today's standards would seem small for even one person. Air conditioning was unheard of in these times, and indoor plumbing was uncommon.

With so many people living and working in the cities, disease and sickness could easily spread. The health of the people and society was deteriorating.

Health care options were limited. Employers did not provide health insurance. Government programs such as Medicare and Medicaid were unthinkable. Communities and charities provided health care to those who could not afford it. With more people getting sick and injuries more common, a need arose for more hospitals, hospices and clinics.

This was the very beginning of the modern health care system. Caring for the public by the public became an important responsibility. However, something had to be done about the conditions of society — *public health.*

The goal of public health was to make people healthier by having clean and habitable communities. Today, clean water, indoor plumbing and garbage collection are taken for granted. In the late 1800s and early 1900s getting sewage and garbage off the streets was one of the first steps to improving the overall health of a community. A safe water supply was an important advance in public health.

A mixture of laws and technological changes slowly improved life at work and at home. Modern medicine was also beginning to take shape. For example, Johns Hopkins Medical School was formed in the 1890s to teach modern medical procedures and offer care to the poor in Baltimore.

Society was changing and so was health care. For the first time a national health care system was emerging. The foundation of this system — an infrastructure — was established. In the early decades of the 20th century health care increased in scope and improved in quality.

During this time, health boards in large cities like New York took an active role in the health of the community. Efforts such as giving children clean milk in school became important programs. Charities, state governments and cities paid most of the costs for health care and community care.

Then, the Great Depression struck America. With one out of every four Americans out of a job, the federal government took a more active role in society. The federal government, through legislation such as the Social Security Act, drastically changed the relationship between the American people and the federal government.

In 1946, Congress passed the Hospital Survey and Construction Act that planned and helped finance a network of community hospitals. The federal government began to form a national medical infrastructure.

Back in 1900 when the Industrial Revolution was just beginning, the population of the United States was approximately 75 million people. By 1960 the population had more than doubled to over 178 million people. Health care was forced to expand to meet the needs of the nation.

Medical technology progressed at an amazing pace. Public health programs were now a major part of society.

BEYOND MEDICINE TO A HEALTHY SOCIETY

However, problems still remained. As the quality of care improved, the cost of health care also increased. The elderly and needy were the most affected by the price of modern medicine.

In 1965, President Lyndon Johnson signed into law legislation forming Medicare and Medicaid. Paying for the care of senior citizens and the needy changed from a local, state and private responsibility to a federal responsibility. The American health care system was fundamentally transformed.

This book has discussed the problems and strengths of Medicare and Medicaid. There is no doubt that these programs are important. The major problem is the runaway cost of the programs. They are victims of not only a costly health care system, but of a society that has drastically changed.

It has been three decades since Medicare and Medicaid were enacted. In 30 years societies go through many changes. For example, in only three decades the United States emerged from the Great Depression, won World War II, and put a man on the moon.

However, time and the changes it brings do not necessarily improve society. A century ago communities were much more important than they are today. Individuals made sacrifices for the good of their communities and their nation. The United States was growing and thriving.

Today, America continues to succeed, but there are many problems that must be overcome. Many of our successes have resulted in new problems. As the nation and society change, solving these problems becomes much more difficult.

Every year another technological marvel improves the quality of health care. Medicare and Medicaid have been expanded to bring health care to more Americans. As a result, many more Americans are now healthy. Since 1965 the average life expectancy in the United States has increased from 70 years to more than 75 years.

As a society our nation is still suffering in many aspects. Since 1965 the violent crime rate has risen from 160 incidents per 100,000 people to 746 incidents per 100,000 people in 1993. In the same time the murder rate has almost doubled.

Since only 1980 the federal government has spent more than $2.2 *trillion* on various health care programs. All of this money has not necessarily resulted in a healthier society. America's inner cities are a prime example.

Many of the gains we are making in health care are being wiped out by senseless crimes. The United States has the best hospitals and doctors in the world. **BUT WHAT GOOD IS THE BEST HEALTH CARE IN THE WORLD TO A CHILD WHO IS KILLED IN A DRIVE-BY SHOOTING?**

Crime is a factor that contributes to a decline in public health. Shootings and drug abuse contribute to health care costs. There are few other places in the world where a person who has overdosed on drugs can receive first-class health care — paid for by the taxpayers.

As our communities become more ravaged by crime, drugs and poverty, the less healthy our entire society becomes. Government rules and regulations can help to some extent. Nothing will help as much as education and **PERSONAL RESPONSIBILITY.**

Education in and out of the classroom will affect health care. Studies and statistics prove that better education results in healthier lives. Improving and expanding education in America may actually save health care costs.

BEYOND MEDICINE TO A HEALTHY SOCIETY

A high school or college diploma is not enough. Common sense and personal responsibility are also important. **OUR SOCIETY MUST STRESS THE IMPORTANCE OF BEING A VIRTUOUS CITIZEN.** This is the key to rebuilding our communities.

Laws and regulations can help, but they cannot form a strong community or keep one from falling apart. De Tocqueville stressed the importance of associations of people as a reason why America was so great:

> *The American laws are . . . good, and to them must be attributed a large portion of the success which attends democratic government in America . . . on the other hand there is reason to believe that their effect is still inferior to that produced by the manners of the people.*

THE AMERICAN PEOPLE ARE THE ONLY ONES WHO CAN STRENGTHEN AND TRULY REFORM OUR SOCIETY.

Government programs can and will help, but true change must come from the people. **CONSTANTLY LOOKING TO THE GOVERNMENT FOR ANSWERS WILL NOT MAKE OUR CITIES AND STREETS HEALTHIER PLACES TO LIVE.**

Programs such as Medicare and Medicaid prove that the federal government can make a meaningful difference in improving our society. Even though their costs are growing too fast, the programs serve a very important function in our society. This book discussed different ways to control the growth of these programs, but these are only partial solutions.

Medicare and Medicaid are only part of our complex health care system. For years, politicians and policy experts have tried to figure out how to solve these problems.

INTENSIVE CARE

One book titled *Big Government* describes the problems in America's health care system:

> *No other country in the world spends as much money as the United States for the medical care and health of its citizens. And no other industrialized, democratic country is more backward in its system of medical economics.*

> *Federal health operations at present are confused, overlapping, and excessively expensive.*

> *Uninhibited expansion of Federal medical expense involves great dangers and...strong measures are needed to control it.*

Each one of these descriptions accurately describes many of the problems with today's health care system. However, *Big Government* was published in 1949, sixteen years before Medicare and Medicaid were formed.

The problems facing our nation today clearly are not new. Paying for health care has been a problem for years. Instead of patchwork reforms, it is time for new and meaningful reforms. The proposals in this book are not necessarily the only and best answers. The most qualified people in this nation need to design proposals that best suit the American people and the financial resources of the nation.

The federal government has a rare opportunity to show the nation how to modernize a program. **SAVING MEDICARE AND MEDICAID WILL REQUIRE SACRIFICE FROM EVERY AMERICAN.**

The success of any federal reform is dependent upon the people of this nation. Sacrificing today to improve tomorrow is the basis of the American Dream.

BEYOND MEDICINE TO A HEALTHY SOCIETY

Individuals must take the responsibility to help others and their community.

Remember, the government represents the owners — the people.

If the people do not have an interest in their community.and their nation, their communities and nation lose interest in them.

Reforming just Medicare and Medicaid will not be enough. The entire health care system must also be strengthened. Most importantly, the overall health of our families, cities and nation must be improved. This can only be accomplished by strengthening the public health.

EVERY AMERICAN MUST HAVE THE VISION AND GOAL OF A *HEALTHY SOCIETY*.

Acknowledgments

This book is dedicated to the men and women who have dedicated their lives to medical research. Our lives have been infinitely improved by their work, which largely goes unnoticed. Thank you for your dedication.

●　　　　●　　　　●　　　　●

This book reflects many hours of research by many people dedicated to educating the American public.

I would like to thank Mike Poss, Drew Moss, Marvin Singleton, Pauline Neuhoff, Bill Fisher, Allison Bishop, Bobbie Van Pelt, and Todd Sharp for their tireless efforts.

A special debt of gratitude goes to Dr. Ron Anderson, Debbie Steelman, and Russell Verney for their invaluable suggestions and ideas.

Ross Perot

Notes

Chapter 3   Beltway Buzzwords

Chapter 4   Medicare: A Growth Industry

Chapter 5   Medicare Part A: Bankrupt in 2002

Chapter 6   Medicare Part B: Problems to Solve

93   **Medicare Part B has grown:** "The 1995 Annual Report of the Board of Trustees of the Federal Supplementary Medical Insurance Trust Fund," (hereafter called Trustees' Report), U.S. Government Printing Office, Washington, D.C., 1995, pp.9-10.

93   **In the last five years:** Trustees' Report, p.10.

93   **Medicare Part B spending:** Trustees' Report, p.10.

93   **Part B now spends:** Trustees' Report, p.12.

94   **At its current rate of growth:** Trustees' Report, pp. 9-10.

100   **"MEDICARE Part B: 1995" Table:** Health Care Financing Administration, "Your Medicare Handbook 1995," U.S. Government Printing Office, Washington, D.C., 1995, p.13.

103   **In 1966, Medicare Part B participants:** Congressional Budget Office, *Reducing the Deficit: Spending and Revenue Options*, (hereafter called CBO), Washington, D.C., February 1995, p.288.

105   **For example, by the year 2030:** Deborah Steelman, Testimony before the Senate Budget Committee, Washington D.C., May 3, 1995.

Chapter 7   Medicare: Solving the Problems

108   **If we don't fix Medicare:** John Kasich, Chairman, House Budget Committee, The Wall Street Journal, April 27, 1995.

108   **One thing is for certain:** June O'Neill, Testimony before the Ways and Means Committee, Washington, D.C., April 2, 1995.

108   **It is not a new issue:** David Walker, Testimony before the Ways and Means Committee, Washington, D.C., April 2, 1995.

111   **The deductible was set:** CBO, p.283.

111   **As unbelievable as it seems:** Calculated from data in CBO, p.283.

111   **Since 1970 the amount spent:** Calculated from data in CBO, p.283.

111   **In 1995, the deductible accounts:** CBO, p.283.

112   **The CBO suggests increasing:** CBO, p.283.

Chapter 8   Medicaid: The Last Safety Net

129   **One out of every four:** Kaiser Commission on the Future of Medicaid, *Medicaid: A Program in Transition*, (hereafter called Kaiser), March 14, 1995.

129   **One-third of all births:** Kaiser.

133   **For example, in May 1995:** Press release from U.S. House of Representatives Committee on Commerce, June 15, 1995.

134   **For about three million senior citizens:** Kaiser.

135   **Nursing homes receive:** Kaiser.

135   **Nursing homes cost:** Health Care Financing Administration, 1993.

137   **In 1993, New York received:** Kaiser Commission on the Future of Medicaid, *Health Needs and Medicaid Financing: State Facts*, April 1995, pp.72-73.

140   **One example is from Louisiana:** Baton Rouge Capital City Press and Sunday Advocate, January 22, 1995.

141   **In one state:** *Medicaid Drug Fraud: Federal Leadership Needed to Reduce Program Vulnerabilities*, (hereafter called Drug Fraud), U.S. General Accounting Office, Washington, D.C., August 1993, p.5.

141   **A nationwide health care:** "Around Texas and Southwest," Dallas Morning News, June 28, 1995, p.28A.

141   **After non-emergency transportation:** BNA Health Care Daily, February 15, 1994.

143   **These trips cost the taxpayers:** Seattle Times, October 31, 1994.

144   **Some studies show that at least 40 percent:** *Medicaid Source Book: Background Data and Analysis*, Congressional Research Service, U.S. Government Printing Office, Washington, D.C., January 1993, p.1093.

Chapter 9   Medicaid Reform: Solving the Puzzle

148   **For example, a study of six urban:** National Association of Community Health Centers, Inc., *America's Health Centers: Value in Health Care*, Washington, D.C., May 1995, p.2.

149   **This voucher system would:** Michael Tanner, "Medicaid Needs a Private Solution," The Detroit News, July 8, 1994.

154   **As of early 1995:** *Medicaid: Spending Pressures Drive States Toward Program Reinvention*, U.S. General Accounting Office, Washington, D.C., April 1995, pp.36-37.

156   **The Tennessee Program:** Stuart Schear, "A Medicaid Miracle?" (hereafter called Medicaid Miracle), National Journal, February 4, 1995, p. 294.

156   **The average annual payment:** Medicaid Miracle, p. 296.

156   **The problem is:** Medicaid Miracle, p.296.

Chapter 10   Managed Health Care

162   **In 1994, HMO and PPO enrollment:** "Managed Care Beats Medicare Any Day," Business Week, February 27, 1995.

162   **During that year, the health care costs:** "HMO Performance Review," Group Health Association of America, 1994.

162   **In 1994, the CEOs of some of the largest:** "HMOs: Executives' High Pay Raises Questions," American Political Network Inc. Health Line, April 11, 1995.

166   **As a U.S. General Accounting Office:** *Managed Health Care: Effect on Employers' Costs Difficult to Measure*, U.S. General Accounting Office, Washington, D.C., October, 1993, p.35.

Chapter 11   Medical Savings Accounts

171   **In 1994, 90% of the company's workers:** Peter J. Ferrara, "More Than a Theory: Medical Savings Accounts at Work," (hereafter called MSA), Cato Institute, March 14, 1995, p.10.

171   *Forbes* magazine: MSA, p.16.

172   **According to the Congressional:** "Are the Uninsured Freeloaders?" National Center for Policy Analysis, August 10, 1994.

Chapter 12   Beyond Medicine to a Healthy Society

178   **When Alexis de Tocqueville traveled:** Alexis de Tocqueville, *Democracy in America*, Part 1, Chapter 5.

178   **Between 1901 and 1910:** U.S. Bureau of the Census, *Statistical Abstract of the United States: 1994*, 114th Edition, Washington, D.C., 1994, p.10.

182　　**Since 1965 the average life expectancy:** *Analytical Perspectives: The Budget for Fiscal Year 1996,* Office of Management and Budget, U.S. Government Printing Office, Washington, D.C., p.17.

183　　**De Tocqueville stressed:** Alexis de Tocqueville, *Democracy in America,* Part 1, Chapter 17.

184　　One book titled: **Frank Gervasi,** *Big Government: The Meaning and Purpose of the Hoover Commission Report,* **McGraw-Hill Book Company Inc., New York, 1949, pp.176, 177, 181.**

APPENDIX A

HISTORY OF MEDICARE Expansion of Benefits (Part A) 1966 - 1990	
Year	**Entitlements and Benefits**
1966	• Persons aged 65 and older who are entitled to monthly benefits under Social Security or Railroad Retirement programs (whether retired or not), or who have specified amounts of earnings credits less than those required for monthly benefit eligibility, or who will reach age 65 before 1968. Not entitled are Federal employees covered by the Federal Employees' Health Benefits Act and most resident aliens. • Inpatient hospital services: semiprivate room, operating room, hospital equipment, lab tests and x-ray, drugs, dressings, general nursing services, and services of interns and residents in medical, osteopathic, or dentistry training: 90-day benefit period. • Inpatient psychiatric hospital care: 190-day lifetime maximum. • Outpatient hospital diagnostic services. • Home health: 100 visits.
1967	• Post hospital skilled nursing facility: 100 days.

APPENDIX A

HISTORY OF MEDICARE Expansion of Benefits (Part A) 1966 - 1990	
Year	**Entitlements and Benefits**
1968	• Inpatient hospital services; lifetime reserve days: 60 days.
1973	• Disabled under age 65 entitled because disability to monthly cash payments for 24 consecutive months under the Social Security or Railroad Retirement programs (excluding spouses and children of disabled persons). • Persons under age 65 who have end-stage renal disease. • Persons 65 or older enrolled in Part B who are not otherwise entitled to Part A benefits, upon voluntary participation with payment of hospital premium. • Services of Podiatric interns and residents.
1981	• Persons who would be entitled to monthly benefits under Social Security or Railroad Retirement program if application were made. • Disabled persons under age 65 entitled to monthly disability for a total of 24 months, not necessarily consecutive, under Social Security or Retirement Program.

HISTORY OF MEDICARE Expansion of Benefits (Part A) 1966 - 1990	
Year	**Entitlements and Benefits**
1981 **(cont)**	• Medicare coverage extended for up to 36 months for disabled persons who disability continues, but whose monthly benefits ceased because they engaged in substantial gainful activity. • Second waiting period eliminated if a former disabled-worker beneficiary becomes entitled again within 5 years. • Home health: Unlimited in year.
1982	• Alcohol detoxification facility services.
1983	• Federal employees. • Hospice: Beneficiary may elect in lieu of other services: up to 210 days. • HMOs covered as providers.
1984	• Employees of non-profit organizations.
1985	• Durable medical equipment provided by home health agencies. • For HMOs clinical psychologists, services.
1986	• Virtually all state and local government employees hired after December 31, 1985.

APPENDIX A

HISTORY OF MEDICARE Expansion of Benefits (Part A) 1966 - 1990	
Year	**Entitlements and Benefits**
1986 **(cont)**	• Liver transplants. • Extends mandatory coverage for all newly hired state and local government employees.
1988	• Home health care ability to leave home. • Disabled persons after a period of employment: Not required to undergo another 2-year waiting time.
1990	• Hospice care is extended beyond 210 days when enrollee is certified as terminally ill.

APPENDIX B

HISTORY OF MEDICARE Expansion of Benefits (Part B) 1966 - 1991	
Year	**Entitlements and Benefits**
1966	• Residents aged 65 and older and persons entitled to Part A benefits upon voluntary participation with payment of a monthly Part B premium. State welfare agencies may "buy in" for public assistance recipients and pay the premiums on their behalf. • Physician and surgeon services: in-hospital services of anesthesiologists, pathologists, radiologists, and psychiatrists; other medical services including various diagnostic tests, limited ambulance services, prosthetic devices, and supplies used for fractures. • Rental of durable medical equipment used at home (including equipment for dialysis). • Home health: 100 visits. • Outpatient mental health.
1968	• Outpatient hospital diagnostic services (transferred from Part A); physical therapy services in a facility. • Durable medical equipment. • Inpatient services of pathologists and radiologists: No deductible or coinsurance.
1973	• Persons under 65 entitled to Medicare

HISTORY OF MEDICARE Expansion of Benefits (Part B) 1966 - 1991	
Year	**Entitlements and Benefits**
	Hospital Insurance benefits upon voluntary participation with payments of Part B premium. • Outpatient speech pathology services. • Prosthetic lenses provided by doctor of optometry. • Home health: No deductible or coinsurance.
1978	• Services in rural health clinics.
1981	• Home health. • Facility costs of surgeries in freestanding ambulatory surgery centers: Limited to certain surgeries. • Outpatient physical therapy. • Comprehensive outpatient rehabilitation services. • Inpatient services of pathologists and radiologists: No deductible or coinsurance when physician accepts assignment.
1983	• HMOs covered as providers of benefits. • Inpatient services of pathologists and radiologists: Subject to coinsurance.
1985	• Pheumonococcal vaccine, hepatitis B for selected populations.

Year	Entitlements and Benefits
HISTORY OF MEDICARE Expansion of Benefits (Part B) 1966 - 1991	
	• Outpatient physical therapy services. • Outpatient ambulatory surgery services of dentist and podiatrist in office. • Services provided by clinical psychologists in HMOs.
1986	• Liver transplant services. • Extend mandatory coverage for all newly hired state and local government employees.
1987	• Vision care services by an optometrist. • Occupational therapy services including services furnished in a skilled-nursing facility, clinic, rehabilitation agency, public health agency, or by an independently practicing therapist. • Outpatient immunosuppressive therapy services: Up to 1 year after transplant; in certain delivery settings. • Ambulatory surgical procedures performed in ambulatory surgical centers, hospital outpatient departments, and certain physician offices: Coinsurance and deductible no longer waived.
1988	• Increases maximum payment for mental health services and includes outpatient mental health services provided

APPENDIX B

HISTORY OF MEDICARE Expansion of Benefits (Part B) 1966 - 1991	
Year	**Entitlements and Benefits**
	by ambulatory hospital-based or hospital-affiliated programs under the supervision of a physician. • Services provided by clinical social workers, physician assistants, clinical psychologists, and certified nurse-midwives: Limited to certain settings. • Home health care ability to leave home. • Disabled persons after a period of employment: Not required to under another 2-year waiting period.
1990	• Limit on mental health benefits eliminated. Coverage extended to services of clinical psychologists and social workers.
1991	• Routine mammography screenings.

APPENDIX C

HISTORY OF MEDICAID		
Expansion of Benefits 1965 - 1991		
Year	Legislation	
1965	**Social Security Amendments of 1965 (P.L. 89-97)** Established the Medicaid program	
1967	**Social Security Amendments of 1967 (P.L. 90-248)** • Limited financial standards for the medically needy • Established the Early and Periodic Screening, Diagnostic and Treatment (EPSDT) program to improve child health • Permitted Medicaid beneficiaries to use providers of their choice	
1971	**Act of December 14, 1971 (P.L. 92-223)** • Allowed States to cover services in intermediate care facilities (ICFs) and ICFs for the mentally retarded (ICFs/MR)	
1972	**Social Security Amendments of 1972 (P.L. 92-603)** • Repealed 1965 provision requiring States to move toward comprehensive Medicaid coverage • Allowed States to cover beneficiaries under age 22 in psychiatric hospitals	

HISTORY OF MEDICAID Expansion of Benefits 1965 - 1991	
Year	Legislation
1977	**Medicare-Medicaid Anti-Fraud and Abuse Amendments of 1977 (P.L. 95-142)** • Established Medicaid Fraud Control Units
1980	**Mental Health Systems Act (P.L. 96-398)** • Required most States to develop a computerized Medicaid Management Information System (MMIS) **Omnibus Reconciliation Act of 1980 (P.L. 96-499)** • Boren amendment permitted States to establish payment systems for nursing home care in lieu of Medicare's rules
1981	**Omnibus Budget Reconciliation Act of 1981 (OBRA 81, P.L. 97-35)** • Enacted 3-year reductions in Federal matching percentages for States whose spending exceeded growth targets • Established section 1915(b) and 1915(c) waiver programs (freedom-of-choice and home and community-based services) • Extended the Boren amendment to in-patient hospital services • Eliminated special penalties for non-compliance with EPSDT requirements.

APPENDIX C

HISTORY OF MEDICAID
Expansion of Benefits 1965 - 1991

Year	Legislation
1981 **(cont)**	• Gave States with medically needy programs broader authority to limit coverage
1984	**Deficit Reduction Act of 1984 (DEFRA, P.L. 98-369)** • Eliminated categorical tests for certain pregnant women and young children
1986	**Consolidated Omnibus Budget Reconciliation Act of 1985 (OBRA, P.L. 99-272)** • Extended coverage to all pregnant women meeting AFDC financial standards **Omnibus Budget Reconciliation Act of 1986 (OBRA 86, P.L. 99-509)** • Allowed coverage of pregnant women and young children to 100 percent of poverty • Established a new category of "qualified Medicare beneficiaries" (QMBs)
1987	**Medicare and Medicaid Patient and ProProgram Protection Act of 1987 (P.L. 100-93)** • Strengthened authorities to sanction and exclude providers **Omnibus Budget Reconciliation Act of 1987 (OBRA 87, P.L. 100-203)**

APPENDIX C

HISTORY OF MEDICAID Expansion of Benefits 1965 - 1991	
Year	**Legislation**
1987 (cont)	• Allowed coverage of pregnant women and infants to 185 percent of poverty • Strengthened quality of care standards and monitoring of nursing homes • Strengthened OBRA 81 requirement that States provide additional payment to hospitals treating a disproportionate share of low-income patients
1988	**Medicare Catastrophic Coverage Act of 1988 (MCCA, P.L. 100-360)** • Mandated coverage of pregnant women and infants to 100 percent of poverty • Expanded coverage of low-income Medicare beneficiaries • Established special eligibility rules for institutionalized persons whose spouse remained in the community to prevent "spousal impoverishment" **Family Support Act of 1988 (P.L. 100-485)**
	• Extended work transition coverage for families losing AFDC because of increased earnings and expanded coverage for two-parent families whose principal earner was unemployed

HISTORY OF MEDICAID	
Expansion of Benefits 1965 - 1991	
Year	Legislation
1988 (cont)	• Mandated coverage of pregnant women and children under age 6 to 133 percent of poverty • Expanded EPSDT program requirements • Mandated coverage and full-cost reimbursement of federally qualified health centers (FQHCs)
1990	**1990 Omnibus Budget Reconciliation Act of 1990 (OBRA 90, P.L. 101-508)** • Phased in coverage of children ages 6 through 18 to 100 percent of poverty • Expanded coverage of low-income Medicare beneficiaries • Established Medicaid prescription drug rebate program
1991	**Medicaid Voluntary Contribution and Provider-Specific Tax Amendments of 1991 (P.L. 102-234)** • Restricted use of provider donations and taxes as State share of Medicaid spending; limited disproportionate share hospital payments

Source: Table prepared by the Congressional Research Service.

Index

Contacting Your Elected Officials

This country belongs to the people.

Contact your elected officials in Washington to let them know your thoughts about Medicare or Medicaid.

Let them know your concerns.

Only you, the people, can assure that the 21st century will be the greatest in our country's history.

To contact the President of the United States

By writing:

By telephone:

The Honorable William J. Clinton
President of the United States
The White House
1600 Pennsylvania Avenue, N.W.
Washington, D.C. 20500

(202)456-1414

To contact your U.S. Senators

By writing:

By telephone:

The Honorable _____
United States Senate
Washington, D.C. 20510

(202)224-3121

To contact your U.S. Representative

By writing:

By telephone:

The Honorable _____
United States House of Representatives
Washington, D.C. 20515

(202)225-3121

UNITED WE STAND AMERICA ENROLLMENT FORM

❑ Yes! I want to JOIN UNITED WE STAND AMERICA.
❑ Yes! I want to RENEW my UWSA membership.
❑ Yes! I want to GIVE A GIFT UWSA membership to the person listed below. *Please give your name, address and membership number in the space provided on the next page.*

Name _____
　　　　　First　　　　　Middle Initial　　　　Last

There is no additional cost for family members residing at the address listed below. Please provide their names on the next page.

Address _____Apt. # _____

City/State/Zip _____

Day Phone　　　(_____)_____

Evening Phone　(_____)_____

Fax #　　　　　(_____)_____

Membership # _____
　　　　　　　(for renewing members only)

❑ Enclosed is my $20 annual fee.　　　　　　　$_____

❑ I would like to make the following
　contribution to United We Stand America.
　❑ $250　❑ $100　❑ $50　❑ Other　　　$_____
　　　　　　　　　　　　　　TOTAL　$_____

❑ Enclosed is a check for the total made payable to: UWSA
　Mail to: UWSA, P.O. Box 6, Dallas, TX 75221-0006

❑ Please charge the total to the credit card below.
　Number _ _ _ _ _ _ _ _ _ _ _ _ _ _ _ _ Expiration Date _ _ - _ _
　Type of card ❑Amer. Exp. ❑Discover ❑Mastercard ❑VISA
　Signature _____
　Contributions and membership fees are not tax deductible.

Please list additional family members who reside at your address to be included on you Family Membership:

Please Print		
Name _____		
First	Middle Initial	Last
Name _____		
First	Middle Initial	Last
Name _____		
First	Middle Initial	Last
Name _____		
First	Middle Initial	Last

Gift Membership Sponsor:

Please Print
Sponsor's Name _____
Address _____
City/State/Zip _____
Member # _____
❑ I am not a member, but wish to give a gift membership.

For more information about United We Stand America, call (214)960-9100.